Colour Atlas of Anatomical Pathology

£19.95

D0493998

	LIBRARY JOHN TURNER BUILDING WARWICK HOSPITAL

TITLE	
A colour atlas of anatomical pathology	

AUTHOR	COPY NO
COOKE, R. & STEWART. B.	001971

CLASS MARK	
QZ 17 COO	

BRB

This book is to be returned on or before
the last date stamped below.   BRB

- 9 FEB 1995

1 3 MAY 2

2 2 JUN 2006

Colour Atlas of Anatomical Pathology

Robin A. Cooke MD DCP FRCPA FRCPath

Director of Anatomical Pathology, Royal Brisbane Hospital,
Brisbane, Australia
Clinical Teacher, University of Queensland, Brisbane, Australia
Visiting Professor and External Consultant, University of
Papua New Guinea, Papua New Guinea

Brian Stewart RBI

Senior Photographer, Royal Brisbane Hospital, Brisbane,
Australia

CHURCHILL LIVINGSTONE
EDINBURGH LONDON MELBOURNE AND NEW YORK 1987

LIBRARY
JOHN TURNER BUILDING
WARWICK HOSPITAL
WARWICK

001971

CHURCHILL LIVINGSTONE
Medical Division of Longman Group UK Limited

Distributed in the United States of America by Churchill
Livingstone Inc., 1560 Broadway, New York, N.Y. 10036, and
by associated companies, branches and representatives
throughout the world.

© Text: Longman Group UK Limited 1987
© Illustrations: North Brisbane Hospitals Board 1987

All rights reserved. No part of this publication may be
reproduced, stored in a retrieval system, or transmitted in any
form or by any means, electronic, mechanical, photocopying,
recording or otherwise, without the prior permission of the
publishers (Churchill Livingstone, Robert Stevenson House,
1–3 Baxter's Place, Leith Walk, Edinburgh EH1 3AF).

First published 1987

ISBN 0-443-03596-2

British Library Cataloguing in Publication Data
Cooke, Robin A.
    Colour atlas of anatomical pathology.
    1. Pathology
    I. Title   II. Stewart, Brian
    616.07   RB111

Library of Congress Cataloging in Publication Data
Cooke, Robin A.
    Colour atlas of anatomical pathology.

    Includes index.
    1. Anatomy, Pathological—Atlases.   I. Stewart,
Brian, RBI.   II. Title. [DNLM: 1. Pathology—atlases.
QZ 17 C773c]
RB33.C64   1987   616.07′022′2   87-8049

Produced by Longman Group (FE) Limited
Printed in Hong Kong

Preface

There are many good student textbooks of Pathology and many good colour atlases of microscopic Pathology. We hope to supplement this material with an Atlas that contains good examples of conditions mentioned in most textbooks and illustrated by colour photographs of fresh, unfixed tissue rather than by black and white photographs or photographs of fixed specimens. The text is confined to a brief clinical history with sometimes a short reference to the salient features of the pathology.

Macroscopic Pathology is learnt by seeing examples of the various pathological conditions in the operating theatre, post mortem room or in a pathology museum. Most undergraduate and postgraduate instruction is based on formalin fixed specimens because this is the most convenient method of preserving them and being able to provide examples of the pathology to be discussed, at times when discussion and teaching are scheduled.

Various methods are used for keeping fixed specimens in a state readily available for teaching. The traditional one is to keep them in liquid fixative in perspex or glass containers in a pathology museum. Museum specimens have a number of disadvantages. They vary in quality from one museum to another depending on the skill and dedication of the prosector and the museum technologist, and on the amount of maintenance done. No matter how carefully the fixation and preparation is done, the colour of the original living tissue is not maintained and ultimately the specimens all become varying shades of grey.

Pathology museums are expensive to establish and to maintain, and many Medical Schools no longer use this method of teaching. In some countries it is difficult to get post mortem specimens which are so necessary for the establishment of a museum, and not every Medical School has a good photographic service. We hope this Atlas will help to supplement the teaching in these situations, too.

Not all of our photographs are of unfixed specimens because some pathological conditions of, for example, brain and lung, are best examined after fixation, and some conditions such as Tuberculosis are handled more safely after fixation.

We believe that the study of Pathology should not be divorced from that of Clinical Medicine, and for this reason we have included a number of clinical photographs to emphasise the importance of clinico-pathological correlation.

We hope the Atlas will be used by undergraduate and by postgraduate students alike, and that it will be useful to practising doctors in any specialty that requires a knowledge of Anatomical Pathology.

We have consciously omitted a chapter on Skin because we consider that this is best illustrated by a combination of clinical photographs and photomicrographs, and there are a number of good texts on this topic.

Brisbane   R.A.C.
1987   B.S.

Acknowledgements

The vast majority of the photographs in this Atlas are from the teaching resource of the Pathology Department of the North Brisbane Hospitals Board which services the Royal Brisbane, Royal Children's and Royal Women's Hospitals. This resource has been built up over the past 20 years. All members of the Department and, to a lesser extent, members of the hospital clinical staff during those years, have contributed to it and we thank them for their assistance. We thank especially the following for the use of particular photographs: F. Abadi, R. Aitken, B. Beaven, K. Clezy, A. Davison, C. Furnival, D. Hinckley, A. Jenkins, N. Johnston, F. Leditschke, M. Lloyd, D. Mc. Guckin, H. Manuel, R. Mortimer, M. Neely, S. Pegg, D. Perry-Keene, L. Powell, J. Richens, J. Tyrer and W. Wood.

Professor J.F.R. Kerr, Professor of Pathology, University of Queensland, kindly made the resources of his Department available to us during the compilation of the Atlas, and Doctor J. Gwynne performed the task of proof-reading the original manuscript. We are very grateful to both of them.

We express our appreciation to the North Brisbane Hospitals Board for granting permission for the photographs to be published.

Brisbane   R.A.C.
1987   B.S.

Contents

1

Cardiovascular system

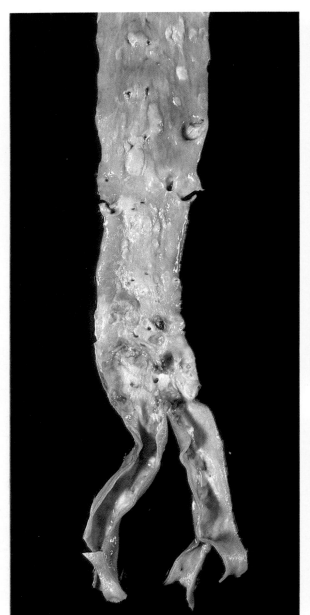

Fig. 1.1

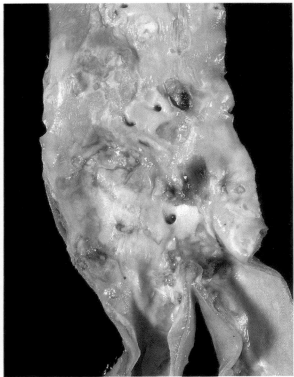

Fig. 1.2

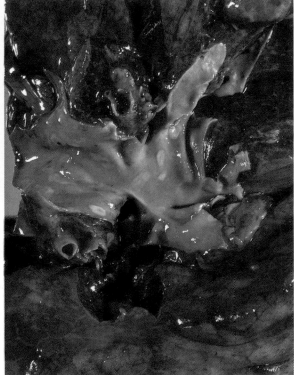

Fig. 1.3

Fig. 1.1 Atherosclerosis. M/51. Atheromatous plaques are present on the intimal surface of the abdominal aorta. 'Complicated plaques' are present in the distal aorta and common iliac arteries.

Fig. 1.2 The same case as Fig. 1.1. Complicated plaques showing ulceration, calcification, haemorrhage and at the origin of the left common iliac artery, thrombus formation.

Fig. 1.3 Atherosclerosis in the pulmonary arteries. F/32. This patient had primary pulmonary hypertension. Significant amounts of atherosclerosis occur in the pulmonary arteries only in pulmonary hypertension

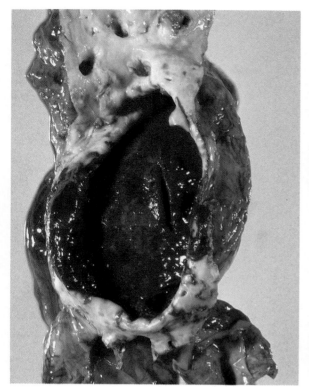

Fig. 1.4

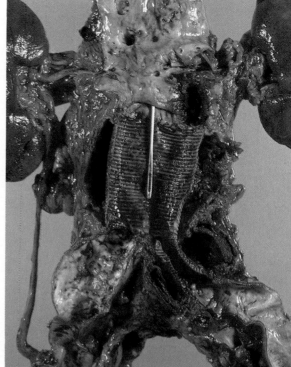

Fig. 1.5

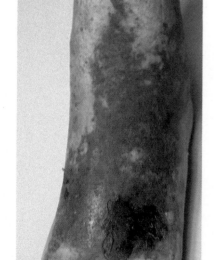

Fig. 1.6

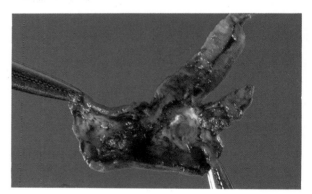

Fig. 1.7

Fig. 1.4 Aneurysm of the abdominal aorta. M/80. The aneurysm is filled with thrombus and death occurred from rupture.

Fig. 1.5 Repaired abdominal aortic aneurysm. M/70. The aneurysm has been repaired by removing its anterior surface (that is de-roofing it), and inserting a dacron graft. The suture lines are all intact. The aorta and the common iliac arteries show severe atherosclerosis. The patient died from a myocardial infarction some days after surgery.

Fig. 1.6 Severe ischaemia of the left foot. M/73. This resulted from thrombotic occlusion of the popliteal artery. The foot was cold and painful. Femoro-popliteal by-pass graft was not successful and the lower leg was amputated.

Fig. 1.7 Endarterectomy specimen. M/73. This area of atherosclerosis has been reamed out of the right common carotid artery at its bifurcation. Endarterectomy is often effective in treating atheromatous occlusions.

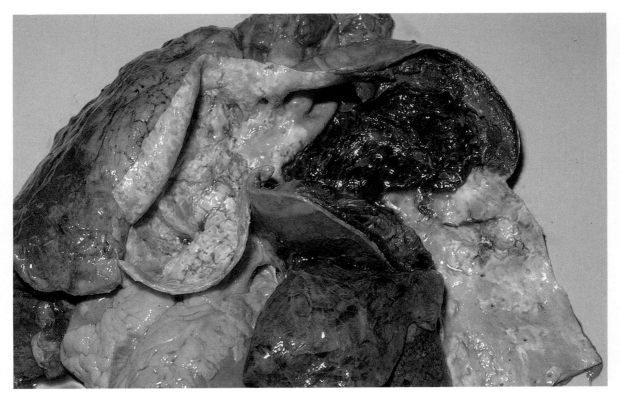

Fig. 1.8

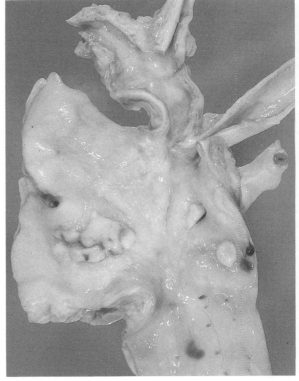

Fig. 1.8 Syphilitic aneurysm of the arch of the aorta. F/73.
The aortic wall is thickened and there are numerous wrinkled,
whitish plaques on the intimal surface. The aneurysm is filled
with blood clot.

Fig. 1.9 Takayasu's arteritis. M/26. A patient from Papua
New Guinea where this condition is relatively common. The
aortic wall is thickened, and there are thick, yellow plaques on
the intima. The walls of the innominate and both common
carotid arteries are thickened and their lumina are narrowed.
The left subclavian artery is almost completely occluded. The
consequences of these occlusions gave rise to the name
'pulseless disease' for this condition.

Fig. 1.9

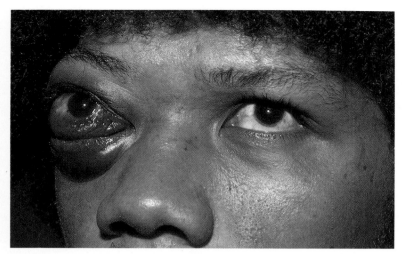

Fig. 1.10

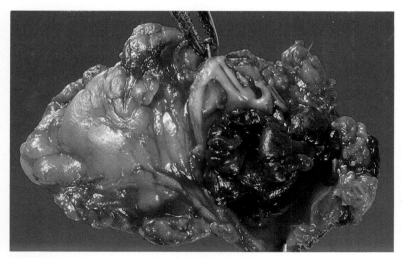

Fig. 1.11

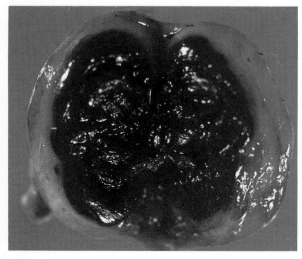

Fig. 1.12

Fig. 1.10 Arterio-venous aneurysm. M/22. This man developed a bulging, red, pulsating right eye following head injury while fighting. The condition developed because of communication between the carotid artery and the cavernous sinus as a result of the trauma.

Fig. 1.11 Saphena varix. F/42. The specimen consists of a 2 cm diameter aneurysm of the long saphenous vein. This lesion presented as a lump in the groin and the differential diagnosis was a femoral hernia.

Fig. 1.12 Traumatic aneurysm of the left superficial temporal artery. M/25. This was treated by local excision of the affected segment of artery.

Fig. 1.13 Dissecting aneurysm of the thoracic aorta. F/73. The wall of the arch of the aorta has split longitudinally and blood fills the false channel. An intimal tear is visible on the lower portion of the aorta. The dissection is extending into the innominate and left common carotid arteries.

Fig. 1.14 Dissecting aneurysm of the abdominal aorta. M/67. The blood has been removed from the false channel and the extension of the dissection along the left renal artery can be seen.

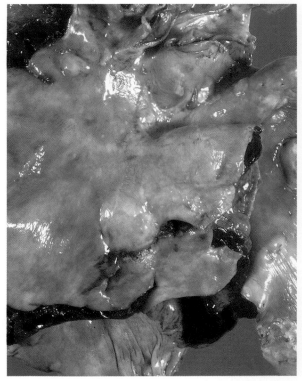

Fig. 1.13

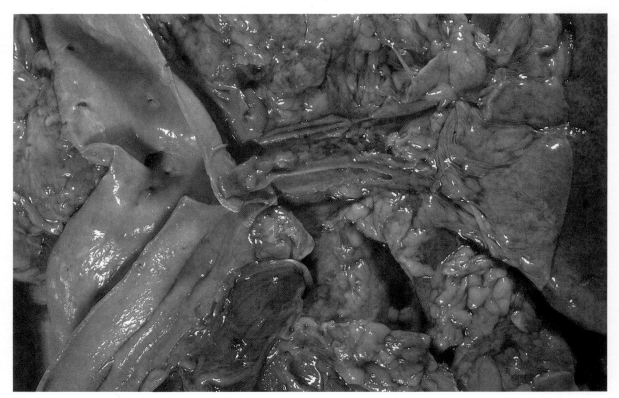

Fig. 1.14

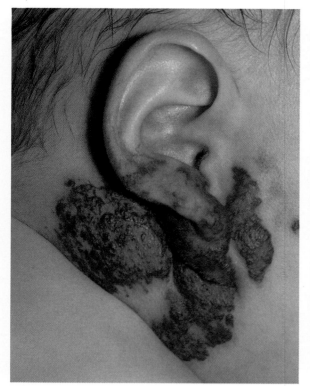

Fig. 1.15

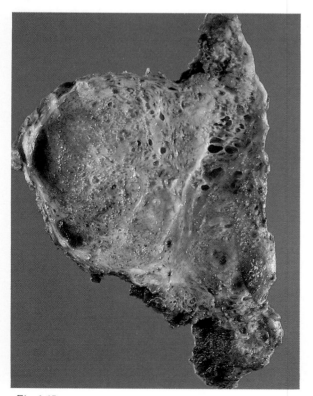

Fig. 1.17

Fig. 1.16

Fig. 1.15 Cutaneous haemangioma. F/3 months.

Fig. 1.16 Lymphangioma (cystic hygroma). M/6 months.

Fig. 1.17 Lymphangioma removed surgically from the left axilla. F/2½. The cut surface shows the spongy appearance of the lymph channels.

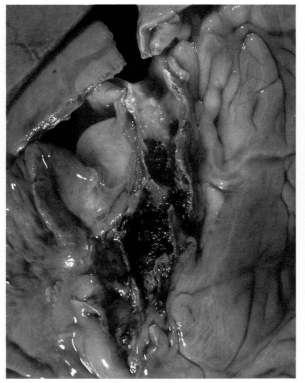

Fig. 1.18

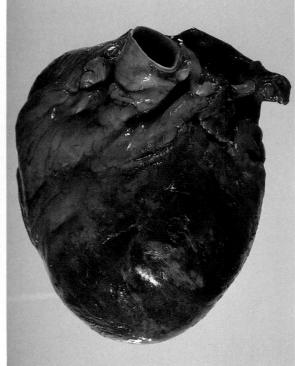

Fig. 1.19

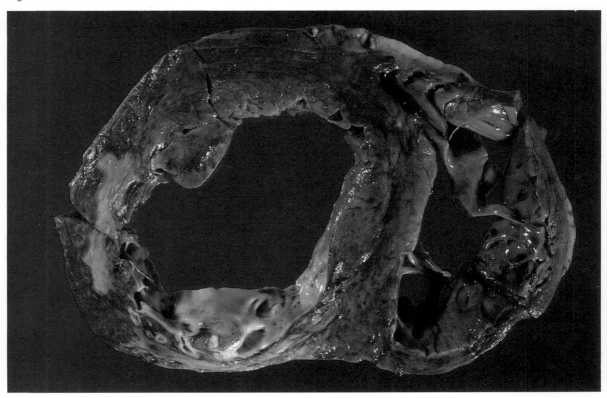

Fig. 1.20

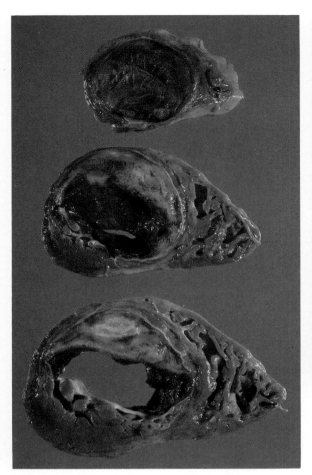

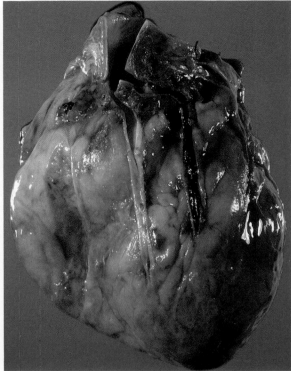

Fig. 1.22

Fig. 1.21

Fig. 1.18 Recent thrombosis of the right coronary artery causing complete occlusion of the vessel. M/40. The coronary artery shows severe atherosclerosis.

Fig. 1.19 Recent anterior myocardial infarction caused by thrombosis of the anterior descending branch of the left coronary artery. M/42. The surface of the heart shows blotchy reddening of the epicardium which is covered by a fine fibrinous exudate.

Fig. 1.20 Old posterior myocardial infarction plus a recent lateral infarction. Posterior view of a slice through the ventricles of the heart. The inferior portion of the left ventricle is thinned and fibrotic resulting from healing of a previous posterior infarction. The lateral wall of the ventricle shows reddening of the myocardium with a yellow area of necrotic muscle in the middle. This is a more recent infarction, probably a few days old.

Fig. 1.21 Old myocardial infarction with mural thrombosis. M/59. The left ventricle is partially filled with thrombus attached to the endocardial surface over the site of a healed myocardial infarction. The patient died from a further acute infarction.

Fig. 1.22 Coronary artery bypass. M/72. The bypass vein has thrombosed. Death occurred from a further infarction.

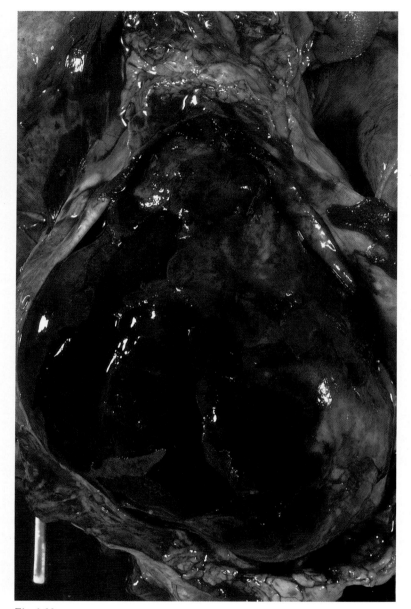

Fig. 1.23

Fig. 1.23 Haemopericardium. F/60. This resulted from
rupture of an antero-lateral myocardial infarction seven days
after the onset of chest pain.

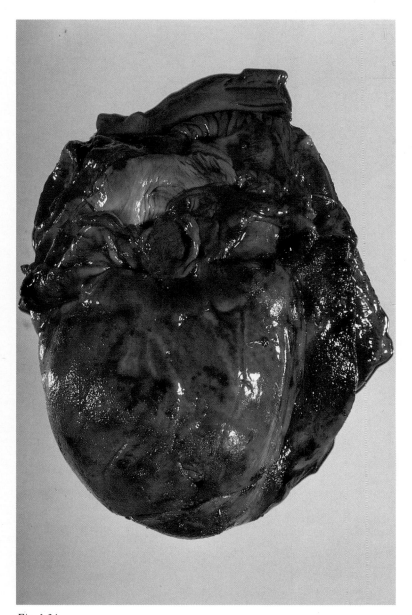

Fig. 1.24

Fig. 1.24 Posterior myocardial infarction with rupture of the ventricle. M/75. The undersurface of the left ventricle shows the features of a recent infarction. At the apex there is a tear resulting from spontaneous rupture of the infarct. This usually occurs about seven days after the acute infarction. Blood escapes into the pericardial cavity causing haemopericardium and death from cardiac tamponade.

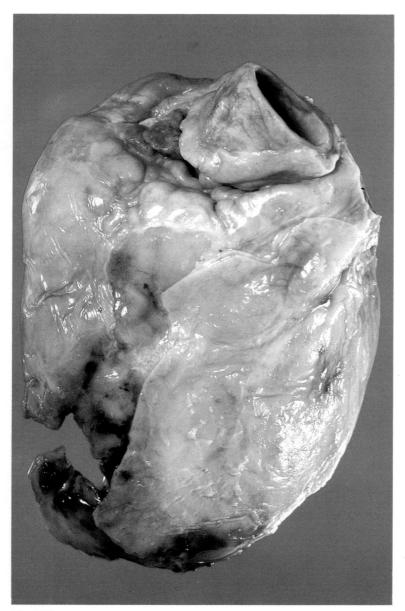

Fig. 1.25

Fig. 1.25 Traumatic rupture of the heart—gunshot wound.
M/30. The apex of the heart has been torn away by the bullet.
The shooting was suicidal and the muzzle of the gun was held
against the chest wall.

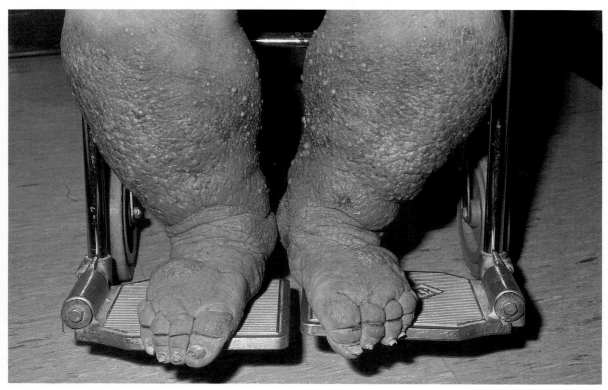

Fig. 1.26

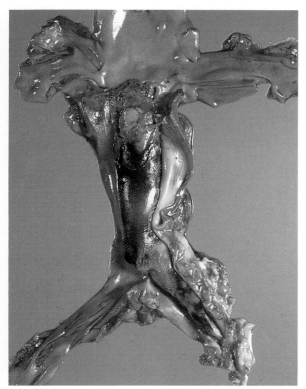

Fig. 1.27

Fig. 1.26 Elephantiasis of both legs. F/76. This condition resulted from longstanding obstruction to the lymphatic drainage from the legs.

Fig. 1.27 Thrombosis of the inferior vena cava and left common iliac vein. F/70. This, too, is a cause of gross oedema of the legs.

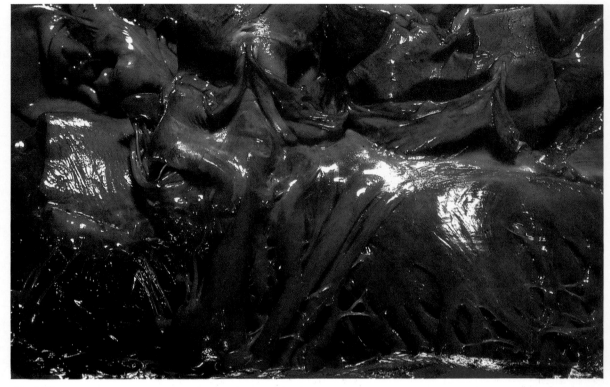

Fig. 1.28

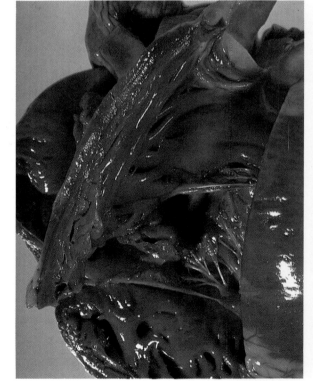

Fig. 1.28 Hypertrophic cardiomyopathy. M/46. The heart has been cut to demonstrate the gross hypertrophy of the left ventricle in the outflow tract. The hypertrophied ventricle bulges into the cardiac chamber below the aortic valve causing a functional aortic stenosis.

Fig. 1.29 Right ventricular hypertrophy. F/32. The heart has been sliced to show the right ventricular myocardium at the outflow tract with the pulmonary valve on the top right. The right ventricle is two to three times normal thickness. Right ventricular hypertrophy indicates the presence of pulmonary hypertension.

Fig. 1.29

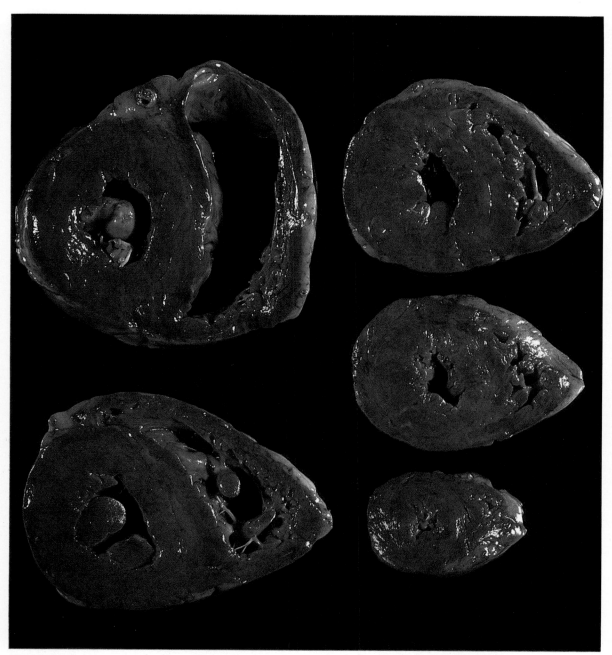

Fig. 1.30

Fig. 1.30 Left ventricular hypertrophy. M/48. The heart has
been sliced to show the whole length of the left ventricle. The
myocardium is grossly thickened. The hypertrophy resulted
from essential hypertension.

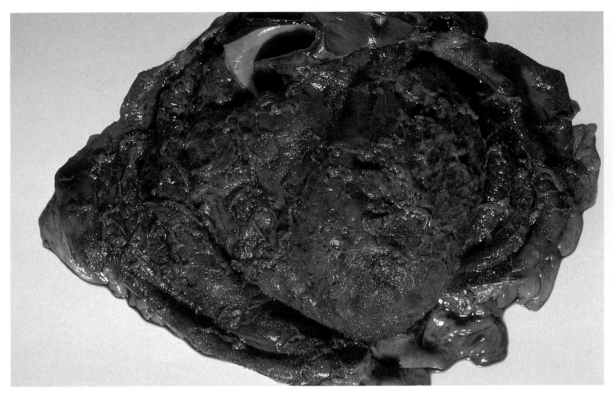

Fig. 1.31

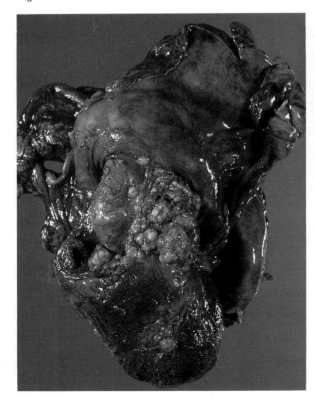

Fig. 1.32

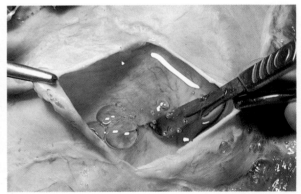

Fig. 1.33

Fig. 1.31 Organising fibrinous pericarditis. M/56. The parietal layer of the pericardium has been separated from the visceral layer with some difficulty. The surfaces of both layers are covered by shaggy, organising fibrinous pericarditis which made the two layers adherent to one another.

Fig. 1.32 Pericarditis resulting from deposits of secondary cancer in the pericardium and myocardium. M/60.

Fig. 1.33 Air embolus. M/39. The patient died suddenly when a large amount of air was accidentally introduced during complicated intravenous therapy. The presence of the air embolus was demonstrated by filling the pericardium with water and making an incision through the water into the ventricular cavity. Bubbles of air then escaped.

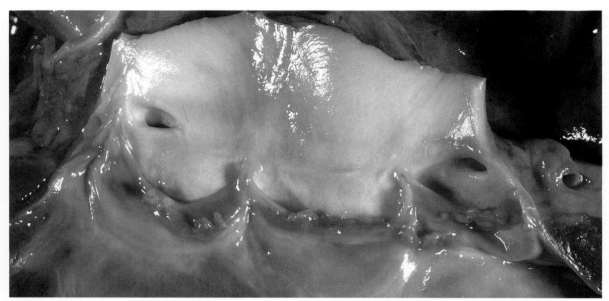

Fig. 1.34

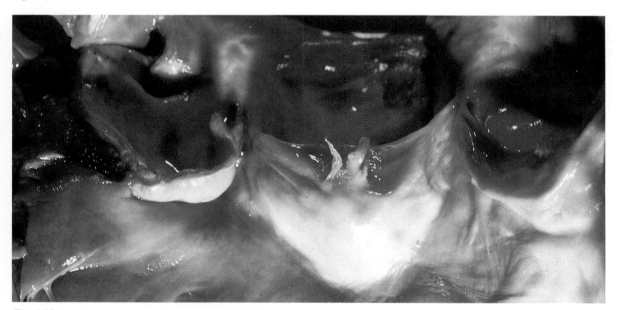

Fig. 1.35

Fig. 1.34 Acute rheumatic vegetations on the aortic valve cusps. F/11.

Fig. 1.35 A Lambl's excrescence on the aortic valve. M/74.
These are aggregations of fibrin covered by endothelium. They must be distinguished from true vegetations.

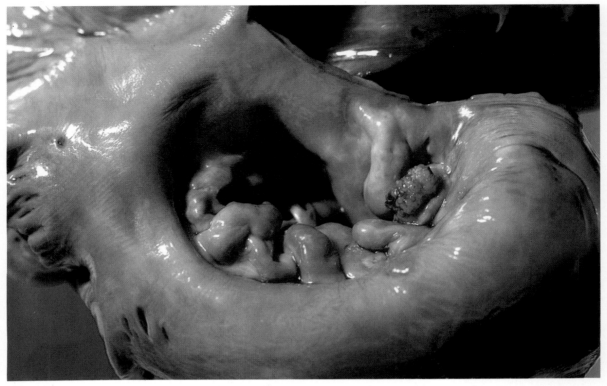

Fig. 1.36

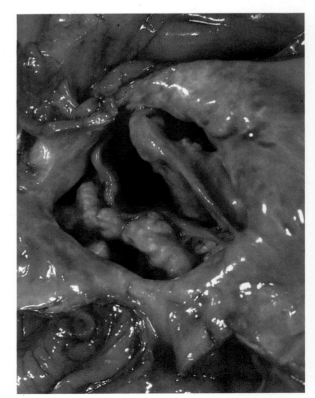

Fig. 1.36 Mitral valve stenosis. F/67. The valve is viewed from the grossly dilated left atrium. The cusps are thickened and adherent, and the orifice is greatly reduced in diameter. The patient had acute rheumatic fever in childhood.

Fig. 1.37 Aortic stenosis. M/76. The valve cusps are thickened, adherent and calcified. There was no history of previous rheumatic fever.

Fig. 1.37

Fig. 1.38 Ball thrombus in the left atrium. M/66. This is a complication of mitral stenosis and auricular fibrillation, and a source of peripheral emboli; however, in this case there appears to be very little abnormality of the mitral valve.

Fig. 1.39 Thrombus in the left auricular appendage. F/85. Thrombus at this site is a complication of auricular fibrillation, and may be a source of peripheral emboli.

Fig. 1.40 Vegetations on the mitral valve in subacute bacterial endocarditis. M/41. These are also a source of peripheral emboli.

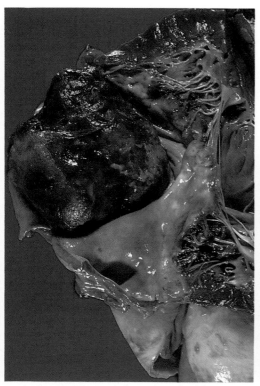

Fig. 1.38

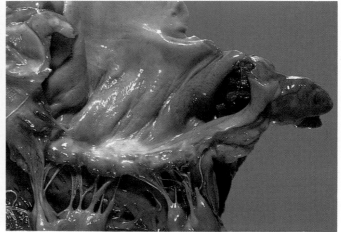

Fig. 1.39

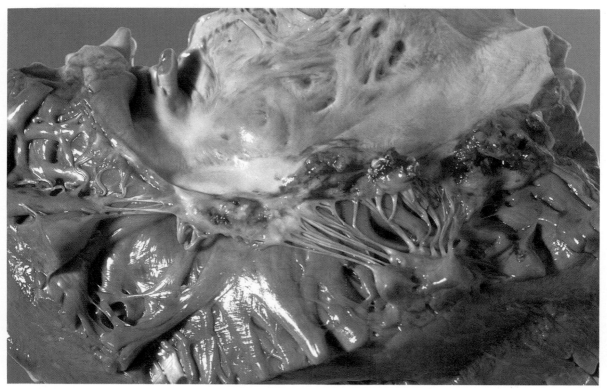

Fig. 1.40

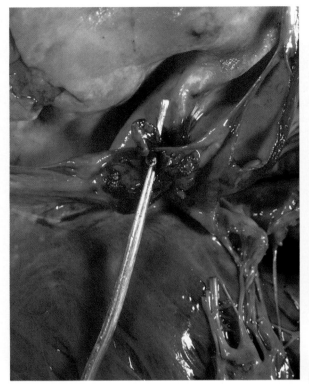

Fig. 1.41

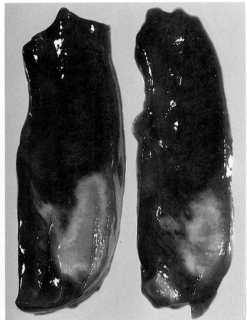

Fig. 1.42

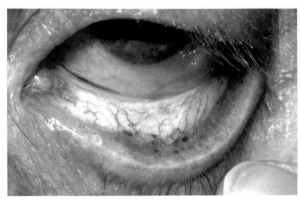

Fig. 1.43

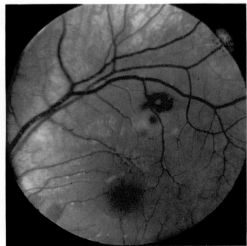

Fig. 1.44

Fig. 1.41 Bacterial endocarditis. Rupture of an aortic valve cusp. M/60.

Fig. 1.42 Recent renal infarct from a septic embolus in bacterial endocarditis. M/56.

Fig. 1.43 Petechial haemorrhages in the conjunctiva from septic emboli in bacterial endocarditis. Note also the linear haemorrhage at the junction between the conjunctiva and the sclerotic. This is another feature of the peripheral embolisation.

Fig. 1.44 Fundal photograph showing petechial haemorrhages from septic emboli in bacterial endocarditis.

Fig. 1.45 Patent ductus arteriosus. F/3.

Fig. 1.46 Transposition of the great vessels. Neonatal death. The aorta arises from the right ventricle and the pulmonary artery from the left ventricle. The pointer is on the ductus arteriosus.

Fig. 1.47 Fallot's tetralogy. M/3. The outflow tract of the right ventricle is viewed in this specimen. There is pulmonary valve stenosis with dilatation of the pulmonary artery beyond this. The right ventricle is hypertrophied and the blue pointer passes from the cavity of the right ventricle into the aorta. This demonstrates the presence of a ventricular septal defect and the fact that the aorta is overriding both ventricles.

Fig. 1.48 Ventricular septal defect viewed from the left ventricle. M/9.

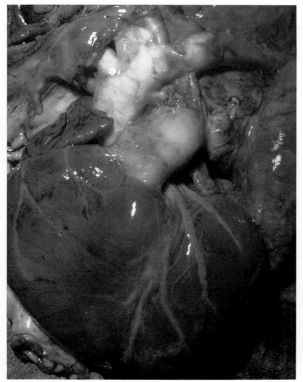

Fig. 1.45

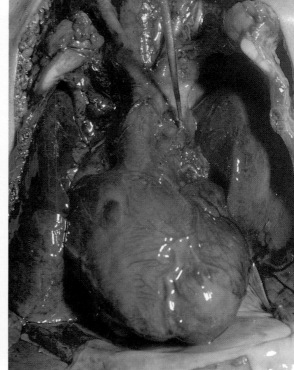

Fig. 1.46

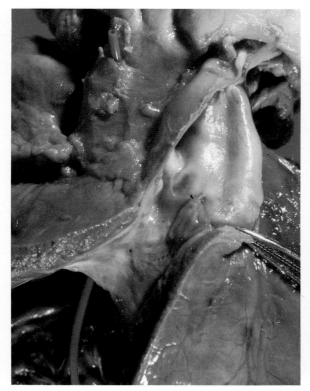

Fig. 1.47

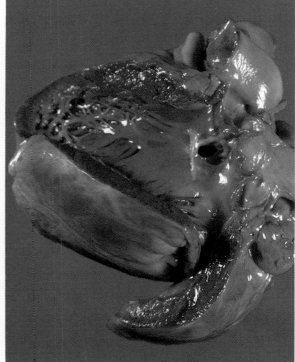

Fig. 1.48

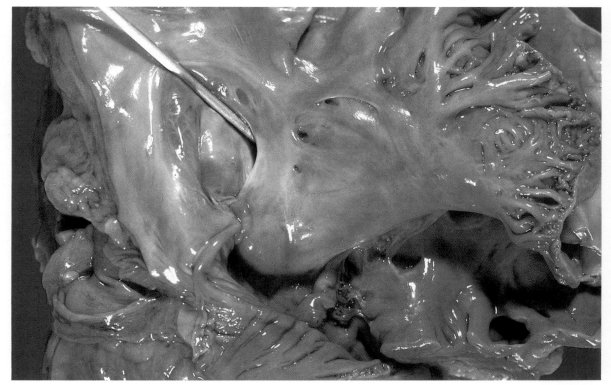

Fig. 1.49

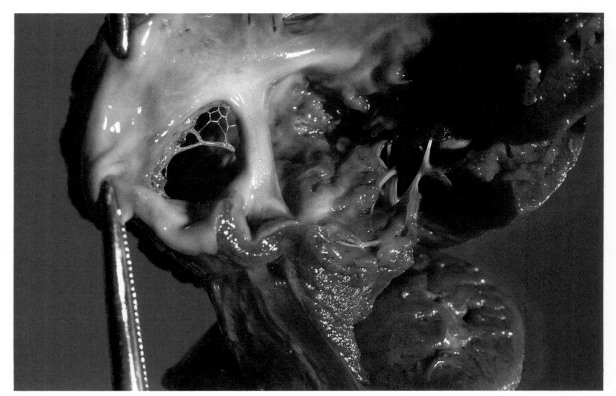

Fig. 1.50

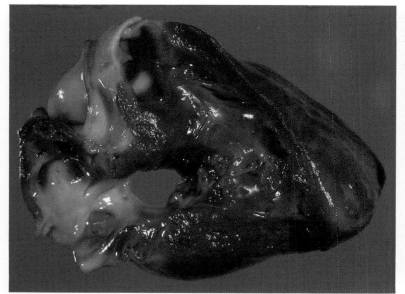

Fig. 1.51

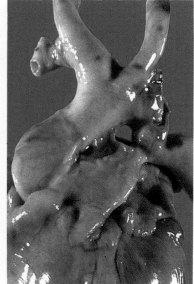

Fig. 1.52

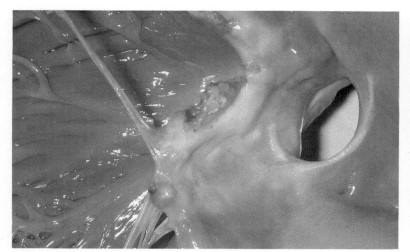

Fig. 1.53

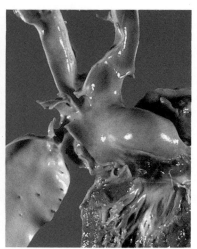

Fig. 1.54

Fig. 1.49 Probe patent foramen ovale viewed from the right atrium. M/70. The foramen ovale is probe patent in a small percentage of normal people.

Fig. 1.50 Patent foramen ovale viewed from the right atrium. Stillborn Down's Syndrome.

Fig. 1.51 Septum primum atrial septal defect viewed from the right atrium. F/4 months.

Fig. 1.52 Co-arctation of the aorta. F/4. The co-arctation is present just distal to the origin of the left subclavian artery (which has been cut off very close to the aorta). The child died from other pathology.

Fig. 1.53 Septum primum atrial septal defect plus a cleft in the anterior cusp of the mitral valve. F/50. This mitral valve defect is often associated with this type of ASD. There is a small vegetation on the abnormal mitral valve.

Fig. 1.54 Co-arctation of the aorta. The same case as Fig. 1.52. The thoracic aorta has been opened from behind to display the co-arctation more clearly.

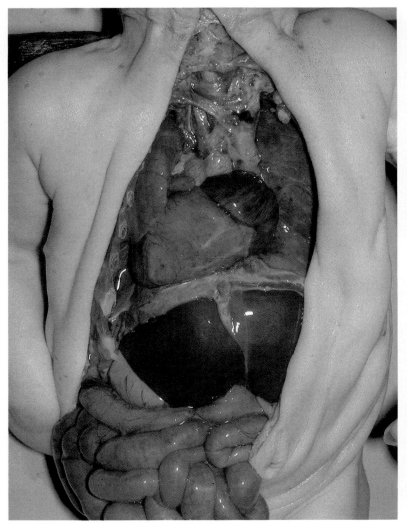

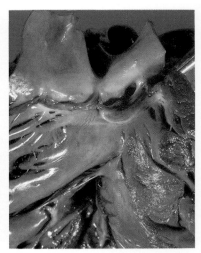

Fig. 1.56

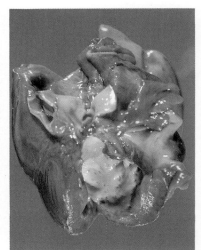

Fig. 1.55

Fig. 1.57

Fig. 1.55 Situs inversus. Neonatal death from respiratory distress. The superior vena cava is on the left, the cardiac apex on the right; the stomach is on the right and the liver on the left.

Fig. 1.56 Left coronary artery arising from the pulmonary trunk. F/7. The orifice of the coronary artery can be seen arising from the sinus above the pulmonary artery cusp on the right. This is the commonest congenital abnormality of the coronary arteries. Death resulted from myocardial infarction.

Fig. 1.57 Fibroelastosis of the left ventricle. M/3 weeks. Death from cardiac failure. The endocardial surface of the left ventricle is lined by a thick layer of white tissue.

Fig. 1.58 Left atrial myxoma removed surgically. M/68. The patient presented with symptoms of left heart failure and signs of mitral stenosis. The tumour was identified during clinical workup.

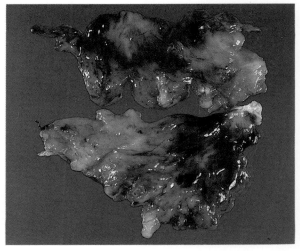

Fig. 1.58

2

Lymph nodes and spleen

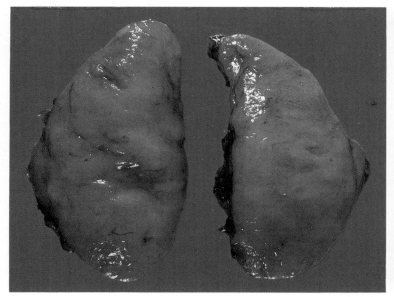

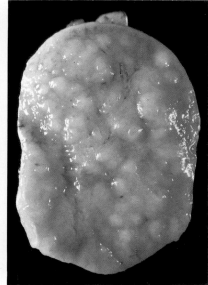

Fig. 2.1

Fig. 2.2

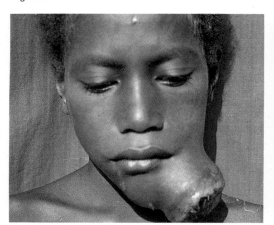

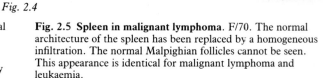

Fig. 2.3

Fig. 2.4

Fig. 2.1 Diffuse malignant lymphoma. M/73. This inguinal lymph node shows complete obliteration of its normal architecture by fleshy, tumour tissue.

Fig. 2.2 Nodular malignant lymphoma. F/33. This axillary lymph node has its normal architecture replaced by tumour tissue showing a nodular pattern. The exact diagnosis of malignant lymphomas must be made by microscopic examination.

Fig. 2.3 Burkitt's lymphoma. M/8 from Papua New Guinea. This lymphoma is a common tumour in children in Central Africa and in children in Papua New Guinea. About 40% of cases present with jaw tumours. It occurs in all parts of the world, but with less frequency than in these two places.

Fig. 2.4 Secondary tumour in a lymph node. F/43. The node is replaced by black tumour tissue. Diagnosis of the type of secondary tumour depends on microscopic examination, but when the tumour is black, it is very likely to be a secondary melanoma, as this one was.

Fig. 2.5 Spleen in malignant lymphoma. F/70. The normal architecture of the spleen has been replaced by a homogeneous infiltration. The normal Malpighian follicles cannot be seen. This appearance is identical for malignant lymphoma and leukaemia.

Fig. 2.6 Multiple infarcts in a spleen greatly enlarged by malignant lymphoma. F/61. The multiple areas of infarction are well demarcated.

Fig. 2.7 Spleen in Hodgkin's Disease. M/34. This spleen was removed during a laparotomy for staging of Hodgkin's Disease. One rounded deposit was found. The splenic deposits of Hodgkin's Disease tend to be discrete and round, rather than a diffuse infiltration as is seen in the non Hodgkin's Lymphomas. This spleen shows early involvement.

Fig. 2.8 A more advanced Hodgkin's Disease than that in Fig. 2.7. F/55. There are multiple rounded, creamy, nodular deposits.

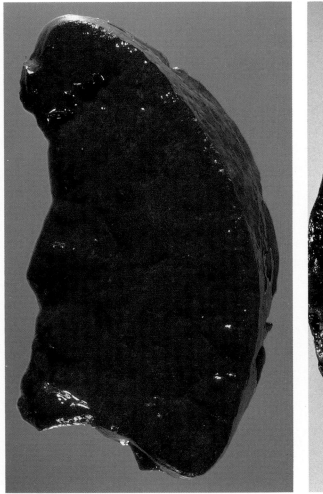

Fig. 2.5

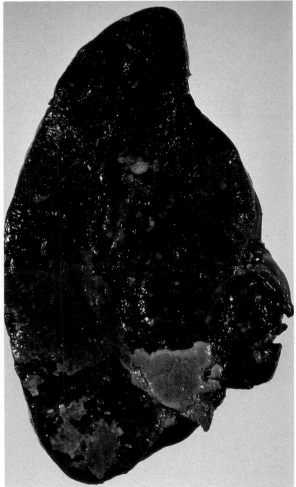

Fig. 2.6

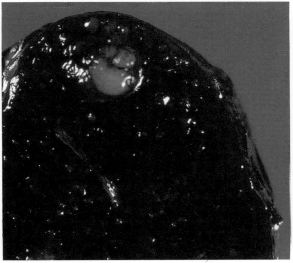

Fig. 2.7

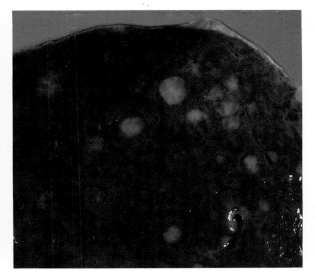

Fig. 2.8

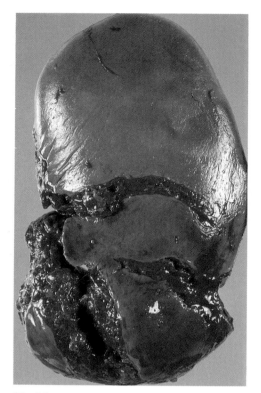

Fig. 2.9

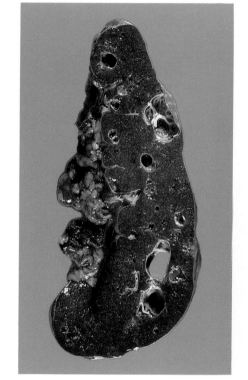

Fig. 2.10

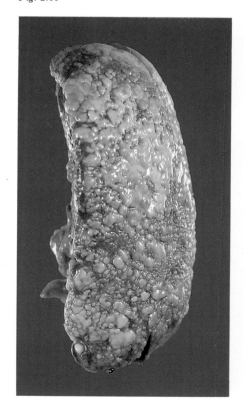

Fig. 2.9 Ruptured spleen. F/16. This was a result of a motor traffic accident. There are multiple tears in the spleen which was removed to stop the haemorrhage.

Fig. 2.10 Simple cysts in the spleen. F/61. These multiple benign cysts were an incidental post mortem finding and caused no clinical symptoms.

Fig. 2.11 Perisplenitis. M/71. The splenic capsule is covered by thick, white, fibrous plaques. This is a fairly frequent incidental post mortem finding. Its cause is not known.

Fig. 2.11

3

Respiratory system

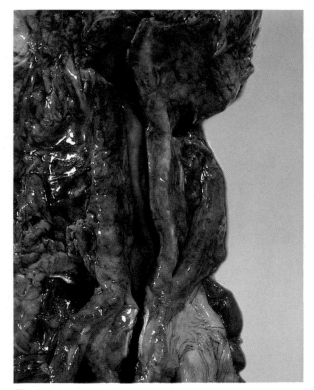

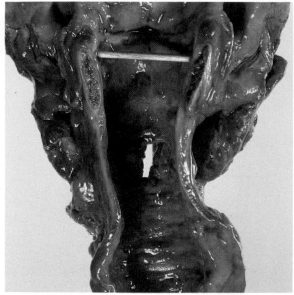

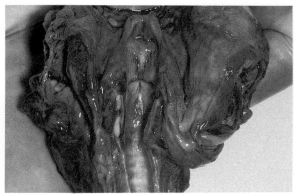

Fig. 3.1

Fig. 3.2

Fig. 3.4

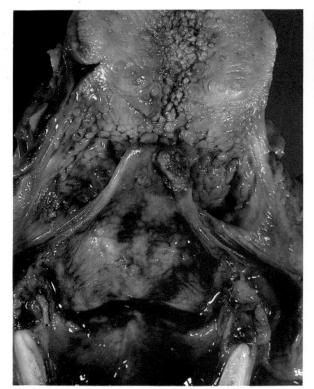

Fig. 3.3

Fig. 3.1 Acute tracheobronchitis. M/68. The mucosa of the trachea is reddened and lined by pus. The patient died of the respiratory infection.

Fig. 3.2 Acute tracheitis associated with the presence of a tracheostomy tube. F/56. The tracheal mucosa is reddened and there is mucosal ulceration and distension of the tracheal wall at the site of the inflated bulb of the endotracheal tube.

Fig. 3.3 Candidiasis of the epiglottis. M/19. The epiglottis is reddened from the acute inflammation, and on its tip there is a green membrane which consisted of purulent exudate plus the hyphal forms of Candida. The patient died from acute leukaemia.

Fig. 3.4 Acute epiglottitis. M/4. This child had a sudden onset of stridor leading quickly to respiratory obstruction and death. The epiglottis is acutely inflamed and swollen, but no other abnormality was found at post mortem. This condition probably has a viral aetiology.

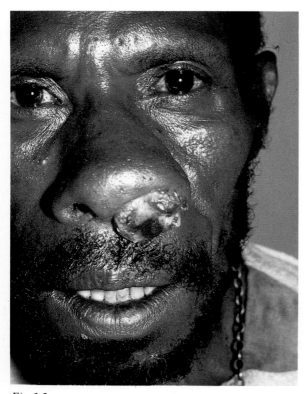

Fig. 3.5

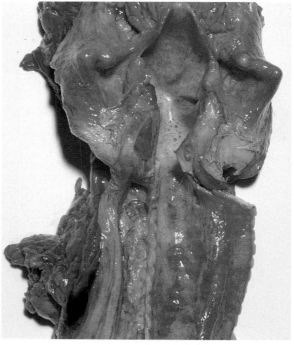

Fig. 3.6

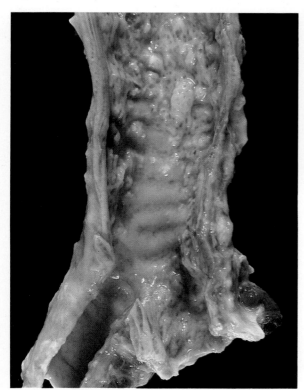

Fig. 3.7

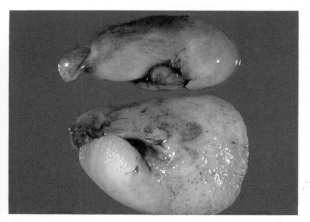

Fig. 3.8

Fig. 3.5 Rhinoscleroma. M/30. Patient from Papua New Guinea. A large mass of granulation tissue fills the nasal cavity and nasopharynx causing widening of the nose. The inflammatory tumour mass is protruding from the left nostril.

Fig. 3.6 Acute pulmonary oedema. M/21. The trachea is filled with frothy oedema fluid. Both lungs were heavy and similar fluid could be squeezed from their cut surfaces.

Fig. 3.7 Tracheopathia osteoplastica. M/70. There are multiple hard nodules on the mucosal surface of the trachea. Microscopically these consisted of cartilage.

Fig. 3.8 Nasal polyps. F/10. These two polyps were removed from the left nasal cavity. Such polyps are fairly common at all ages and are inflammatory in origin.

Fig. 3.9 Squamous cell carcinoma of the hypopharynx. F/65.

Fig. 3.10 Squamous cell carcinoma of the larynx. M/71. The subglottic tumour can be seen in the laryngectomy specimen. The patient presented with hoarseness.

Fig. 3.11 Squamous cell carcinoma of the larynx. M/64. This was primarily an extrinsic carcinoma of the larynx arising in the hypopharynx and compressing the larynx. There is a patch of leukoplakia adjacent to the tumour. Laryngectomy specimen.

Fig. 3.12 Pseudosarcoma of the larynx. M/44. This large, polypoid tumour with a smooth surface is almost completely obstructing the larynx.

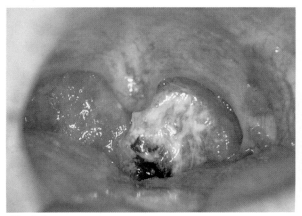

Fig. 3.9

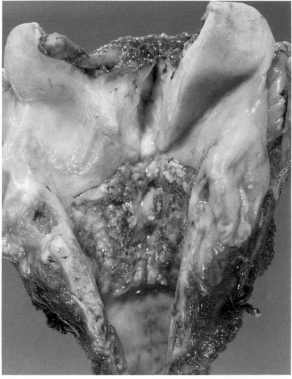

Fig. 3.10

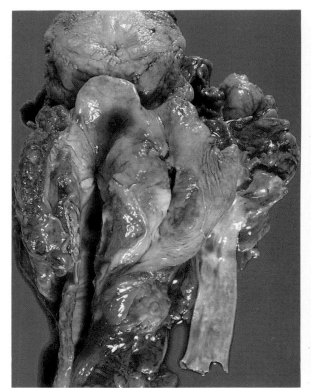

Fig. 3.11

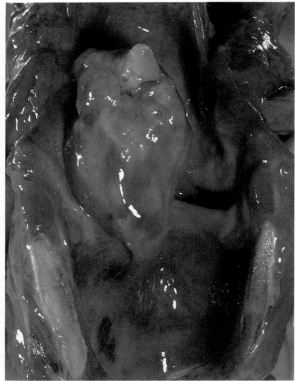

Fig. 3.12

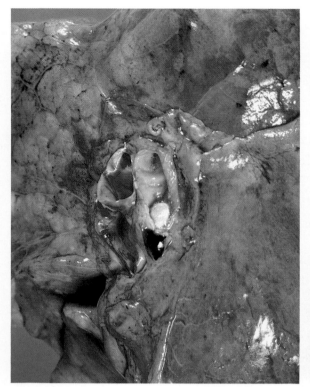

Fig. 3.13

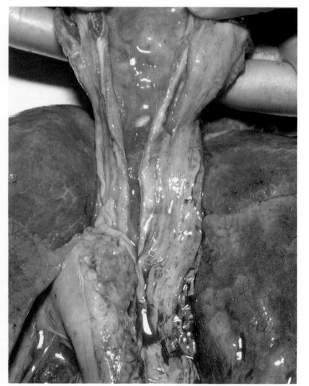

Fig. 3.15

Fig. 3.14

Fig. 3.13 Foreign body (tablet) lodged in the hilum of the right lung obstructing the middle and lower lobe bronchi. M/84. This is the commonest site for an inhaled foreign body to become impacted because of the anatomy of the bronchial tree. Inhaled foreign bodies are most frequently encountered in children about the age of two years.

Fig. 3.14 Unusual inhaled foreign body. M/2. This child was found by his parents covered in his mother's talcum powder. Within a few hours he developed acute respiratory difficulty and died three hours later. The whole of the bronchial tree was filled with thick, semisolid material which could be squeezed out as demonstrated. The powder contained silica and the irritant effect of this must have stimulated the secretion of mucus which in turn mixed with the powder to cause complete blockage of the airways.

Fig. 3.15 Inhalation of vomitus. M/70. The trachea and bronchial tubes are filled with vomitus. This was the final cause of death in a debilitated old man.

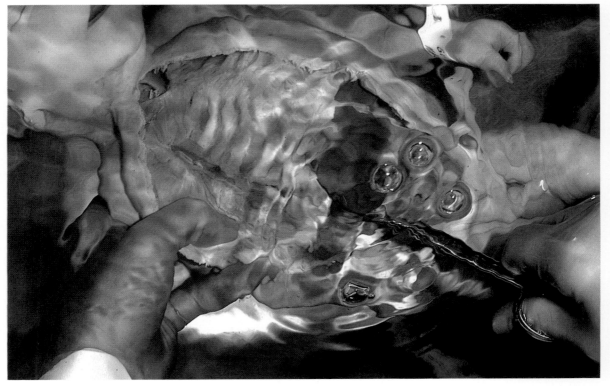

Fig. 3.16

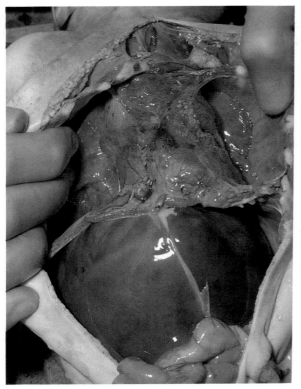

Fig. 3.17

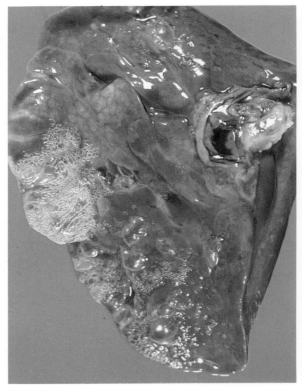

Fig. 3.18

Fig. 3.16 Tension pneumothorax. M/2 days. This resulted from attempts at resuscitation following delivery. The thoracic cavity was opened under water and the escaping air produced bubbles.

Fig. 3.17 Pneumomediastinum. Gas bubbles in the mediastinum of the patient shown in Fig. 3.16.

Fig. 3.18 Interstitial emphysema. F/4 days. This was caused by over-enthusiastic resuscitation following delivery. Rupture of bullae such as these resulted in the pathology illustrated in Figs. 3.16 & 3.17.

Fig. 3.19 Congenital bronchogenic cyst. F/1 month. The child was investigated for respiratory difficulty present since birth; this abnormal cystic area was identified on chest X-ray and was surgically removed from the left lower lobe.

Fig. 3.20 Congenital lymphectasia of the lung. M/10 hours. The cut surface of the lung shows multiple, thin walled cysts. Macroscopically it is difficult to distinguish this condition from interstitial emphysema.

Fig. 3.21 Hypoplastic lungs. F/neonate. Both lungs are hypoplastic, the left more so than the right. The baby had a left diaphragmatic hernia.

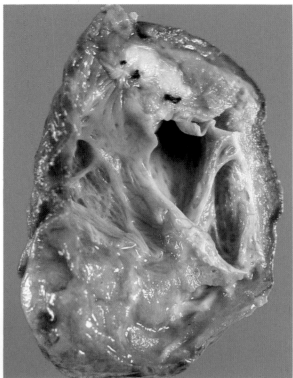

Fig. 3.19

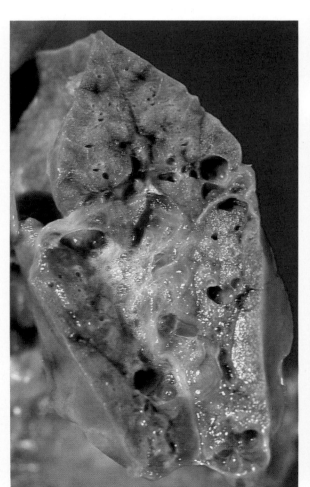

Fig. 3.20

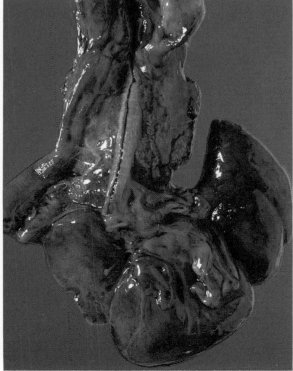

Fig. 3.21

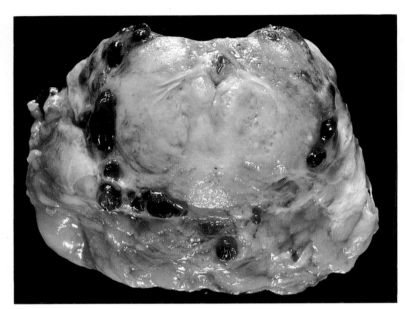

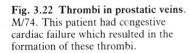

Fig. 3.22 Thrombi in prostatic veins. M/74. This patient had congestive cardiac failure which resulted in the formation of these thrombi.

Fig. 3.23 Pulmonary infarction in the patient shown in Fig. 3.22. This resulted when fragments of the thrombi broke off, passed through the venous system and became lodged in a pulmonary artery. Note the wedge-shaped, haemorrhagic area on the pleural surface of the lung. It is hard, and elevated above the adjacent lung tissue.

Fig. 3.24 Pulmonary embolus. Cut surface of a pulmonary infarct showing the embolus in the supplying artery.

Fig. 3.22

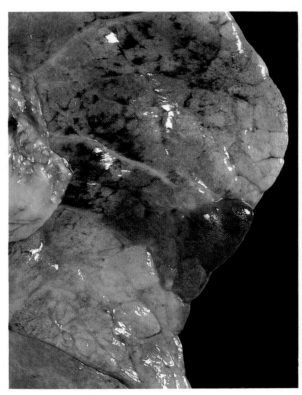

Fig. 3.23

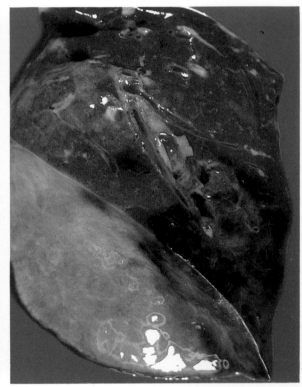

Fig. 3.24

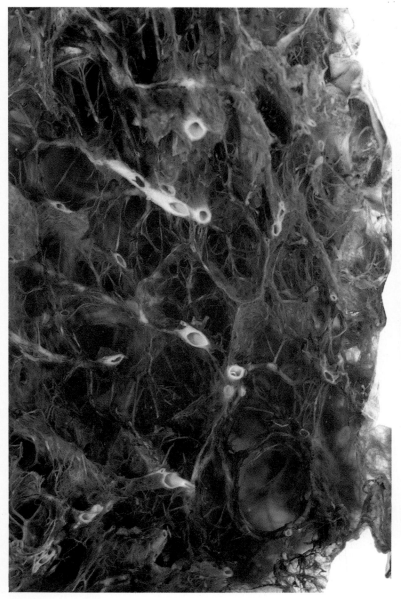

Fig. 3.25

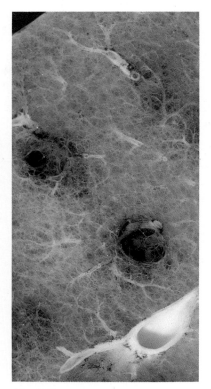

Fig. 3.26

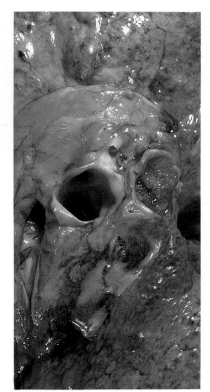

Fig. 3.27

Fig. 3.25 Pan acinar destructive emphysema. M/76.

Fig. 3.26 Centrilobular destructive emphysema. M/70.

Fig. 3.27 Chronic bronchitis. M/69. This man had suffered from chronic obstructive airways disease for many years. Death was due to plugging of his respiratory passages by thick, tenacious mucus shown filling the left main bronchus. The lung itself showed minimal emphysema.

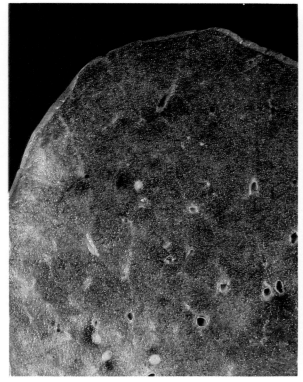

Fig. 3.28

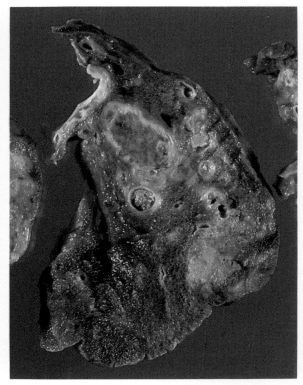

Fig. 3.29

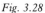

Fig. 3.28 Lung in acute asthma. F/46. The respiratory
passages throughout both lungs were completely occluded by
thick tenacious mucus. This woman had suffered from asthma
for many years and one day she had an acute attack and died.
This sequence of events is well known in asthma and post
mortem examination of the lungs shows the features
demonstrated here.

**Fig. 3.29 Localised area of bronchiectasis caused by
impaction of a mucus plug**. F/49. The patient suffered from
asthma and the mucus plug was obstructing the posterior
segmental bronchus of the right upper lobe. Microscopic
examination showed that the plug consisted of a ball of
Aspergillus mycelia. Mucus plugs associated with Aspergillus
are a recognised complication of asthma.

Fig. 3.30 Bronchiectasis. M/17. Left lower lobectomy was
performed for chronic bronchiectasis. This patient had had
recurrent attacks of pneumonia since his first year of life. The
bronchial tubes are extremely dilated. Their walls are
thickened and fibrotic and 'ribbing' can be seen along the
mucosal surface of some of them. The adjacent lung has been
almost completely destroyed. Surgical treatment of
bronchiectasis is only useful when the condition is localised to
one segment of the lung.

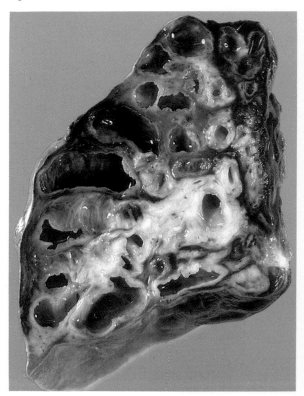

Fig. 3.30

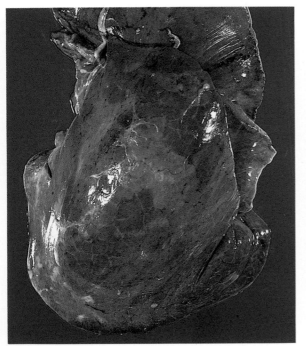

Fig. 3.31

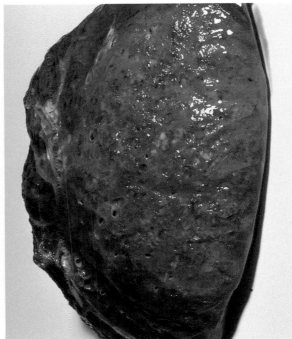

Fig. 3.32

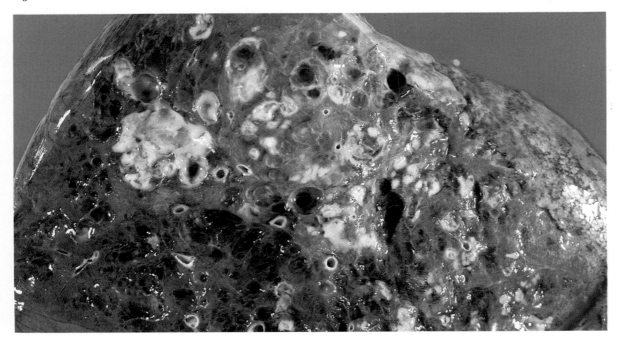

Fig. 3.33

Fig. 3.31 Lobar pneumonia. F/38. One lobe of the lung is consolidated and its pleural surface is covered with a fibrinous pleurisy. The remainder of the lung is relatively unaffected.

Fig. 3.32 Cut surface of lobar pneumonia. M/71. This lung is from another patient but shows that the consolidation is localised to one lobe.

Fig. 3.33 Confluent bronchopneumonia. F/69. As distinct from lobar pneumonia, bronchopneumonia is focal and involves many areas of the lung. The focal collections of pus may become confluent giving rise to small abscesses as demonstrated here. There is no pleural reaction associated with this type of pneumonia. The lung itself is emphysematous.

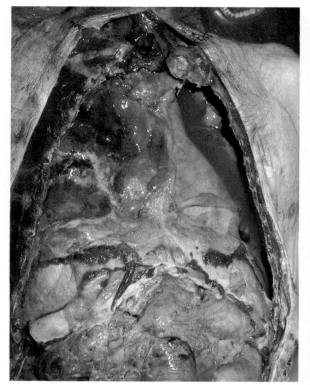

Fig. 3.34

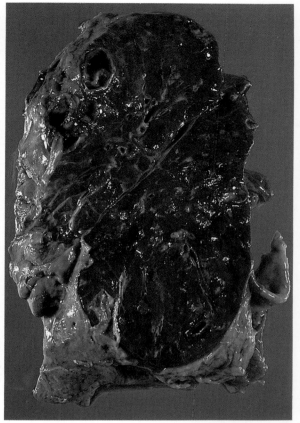

Fig. 3.35

Fig. 3.34 Right sided empyema and left sided pleural effusion. M/68.

Fig. 3.35 Empyema and lung abscesses. M/11. This was a complication of Staphylococcal pneumonia. Abscesses are present in the upper lobe and there is a large amount of pus covering the surface of the lower lobe of this right lung. The visceral pleura is thickened and, posteriorly, some thickened parietal pleura is adherent to it.

Fig. 3.36 Toruloma. M/47. Lobectomy specimen. The lobectomy was performed because an asymptomatic opacity was found on a routine chest X-ray. The cut surface of the lesion is grey in colour and has a rather mucoid appearance.

Fig. 3.37 Miliary torulosis of the lung. F/45. Multiple, yellowish nodules were present throughout both lungs.

Fig. 3.38 Aspergilloma. M/52. The upper lobe of the lung is replaced by a mass of grey tissue. Aspergillus may cause pneumonia which has no distinguishing macroscopic features, but when it forms a large mass like this, it is usually referred to as an Aspergilloma.

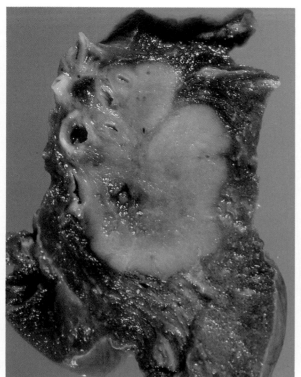

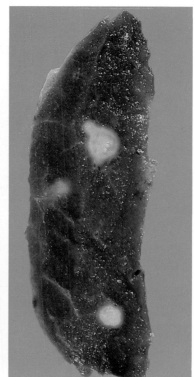

Fig. 3.36   *Fig. 3.37*

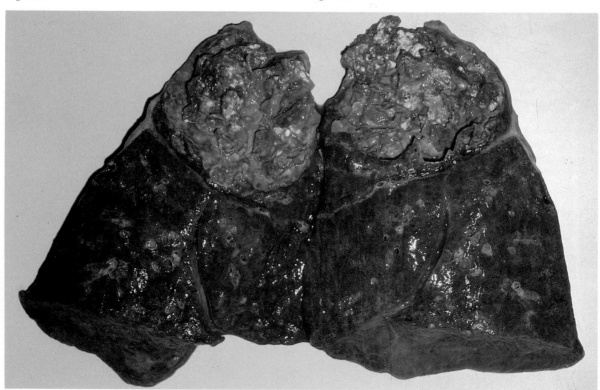

Fig. 3.38

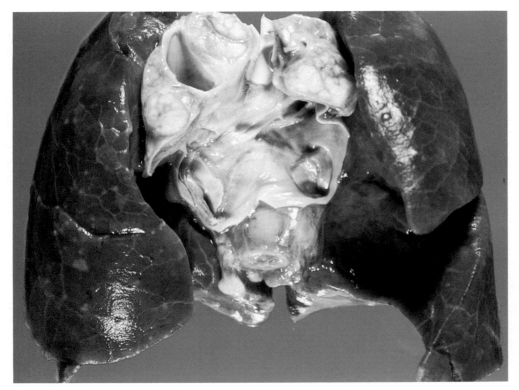

Fig. 3.39

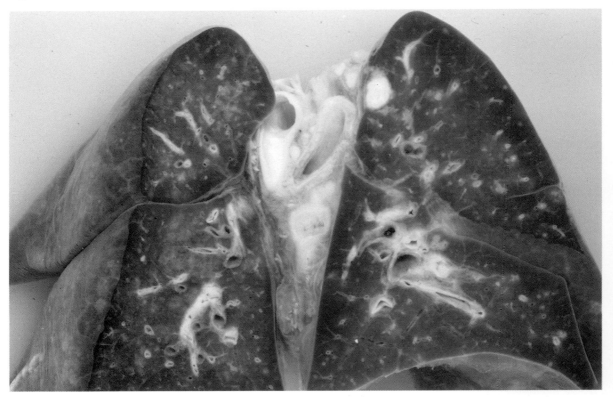

Fig. 3.40

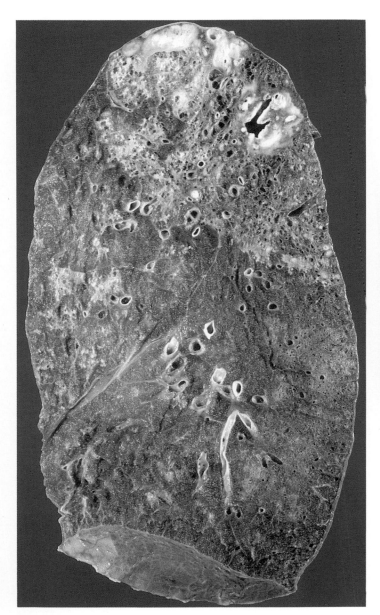

Fig. 3.41

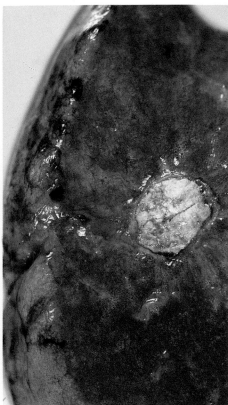

Fig. 3.42

Fig. 3.39 Miliary tuberculosis of the lung with involvement of the mediastinal lymph nodes. F/6. The miliary tubercles appear as subpleural spots.

Fig. 3.40 Coronal section of the lungs and mediastinum from Fig. 3.39. This shows multiple, creamy nodules—the miliary tubercles—throughout both lungs. There is also a large, round, white focus of tuberculous granulation tissue in the left upper lobe just beneath the pleura. This has the appearance of what is called a Gohn focus of primary tuberculosis. The child was moribund on admission and died soon afterwards.

Fig. 3.41 Pulmonary tuberculosis. M/72. The pathology is almost entirely confined to the upper lobe, particularly the apex. There is pneumonic consolidation together with cavity formation. There is also a minor degree of emphysema present. This so-called active adult type of pulmonary tuberculosis was an incidental post mortem finding.

Fig. 3.42 Old, healed, calcified tuberculous lesion in the lung. F/70. This patient had been followed for many years with serial chest X-rays. The lesion had not changed in size, and repeated sputum examinations were negative for acid fast bacilli.

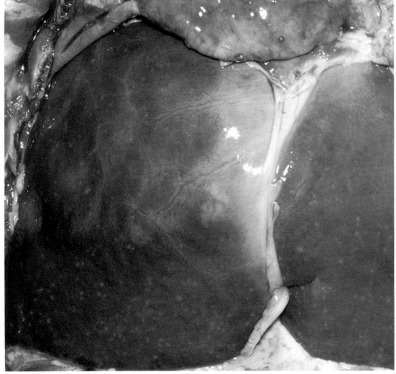

Fig. 3.43

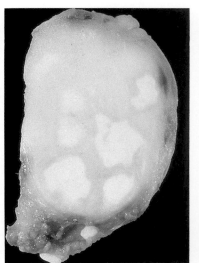

Fig. 3.44

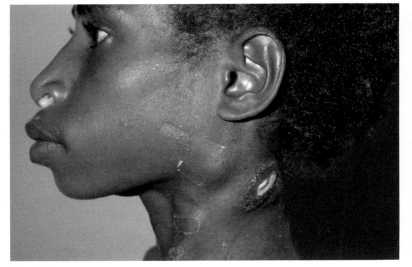

Fig. 3.45

Fig. 3.46

Fig. 3.43 Miliary tuberculosis. Liver from the patient in Fig. 3.39 showing miliary tubercles throughout both lobes. These appear as tiny yellow spots beneath the capsule.

Fig. 3.44 Tuberculous ascites. M/2. In communities in which tuberculosis is common, ascites is a common presentation.

Fig. 3.45 Tuberculous lymphadenopathy. M/14. The boy is emaciated, as is usual with patients with disseminated

tuberculosis. Some of the cervical lymph nodes are enlarged and one of them is discharging through the skin. Cervical lymphadenopathy is a common presentation in communities with a high incidence of tuberculosis.

Fig. 3.46 Tuberculous lymph node. M/24. The cut surface of the node shows its enlargement is due to the presence of many areas of caseous necrosis.

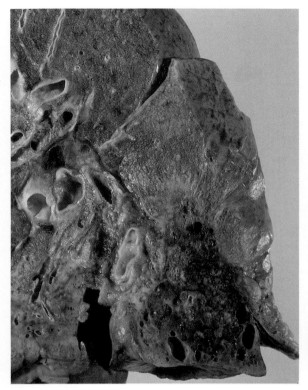

Fig. 3.47

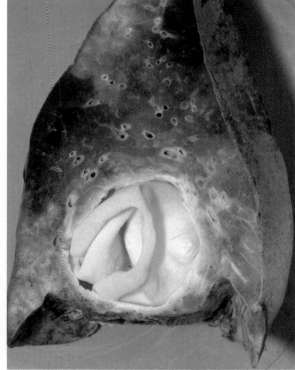

Fig. 3.48

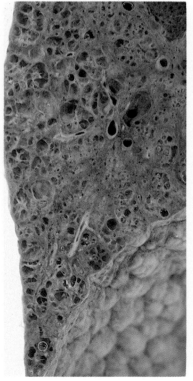

Fig. 3.49

Fig. 3.50

Fig. 3.47 Paraffinoma in the right lower lobe. M/81. There is a wedge shaped, solid black mass in the posterior basal segment of the right lower lobe. Large amounts of oil can be seen glistening on its cut surface. The patient was in the habit of taking a dose of paraffin oil each evening as a laxative. The paraffinoma resulted from small amounts of oil being regurgitated and inhaled during sleep.

Fig. 3.48 Hydatid cyst of the right lung. M/8. The white, laminated membrane is present within the capsule of granulation tissue formed by the host as a response to the Hydatid cyst—a foreign body reaction. This child came from a sheep raising part of Australia.

Fig. 3.49 Honeycomb lung. M/63. The patient had interstitial pulmonary fibrosis, the exact cause of which was not determined.

Fig. 3.50 Subpleural rheumatoid nodule in the lung. M/78. The patient had had rheumatoid arthritis for many years and the lung showed diffuse interstitial fibrosis.

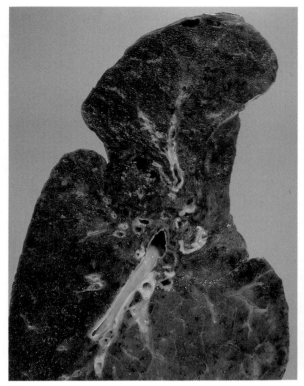

Fig. 3.51

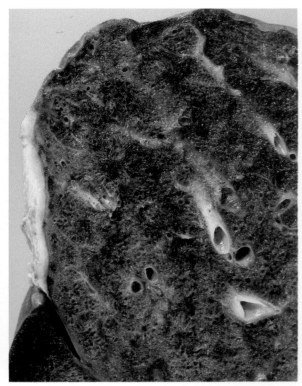

Fig. 3.52

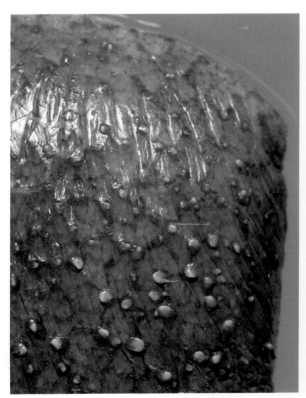

Fig. 3.53

Fig. 3.51 Anthracosis—Coal miner's lung. M/70. The lung shows extensive deposition of black carbon pigment. In the mid portion, the lung has become a solid, black, shrunken mass. This condition is sometimes referred to as progressive massive fibrosis. The patient had been an underground coal miner for most of his life.

Fig. 3.52 Mixed pneumoconiosis. M/77. There is a thick, white pleural plaque attached to the posterior visceral pleura. This indicates exposure to asbestos. The lung shows a heavy deposition of carbon pigment together with some emphysema. This man had worked in an electric power station shovelling coal for about 20 years. In that occupation he would have been exposed to asbestos lagging of pipes as well as to the coal dust.

Fig. 3.53 Silicosis. M/69. Multiple silicotic nodules can be seen under the pleura. This man had worked as a miner for most of his life.

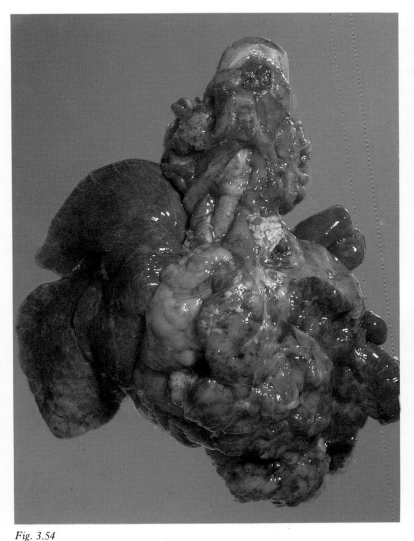

Fig. 3.54

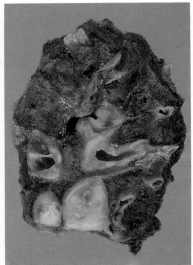

Fig. 3.55

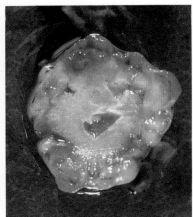

Fig. 3.56

Fig. 3.54 Malignant thymoma. F/1. The mediastinum is filled by a lobulated, irregular mass of creamy tissue. It has extended over the pericardium and caused some compression of the left lung.

Fig. 3.55 Carcinoid tumour of the lung. M/50. Lobectomy specimen. The cream coloured, well circumscribed carcinoid tumour has arisen within the bronchus and caused obstruction distally. The extent of the bronchiectasis caused by the tumour indicates its slow rate of growth.

Fig. 3.56 Benign hamartoma of the lung (Adenochondroma). F/61. There is a well circumscribed, lobulated and hard nodule in the lung. An incidental post mortem finding.

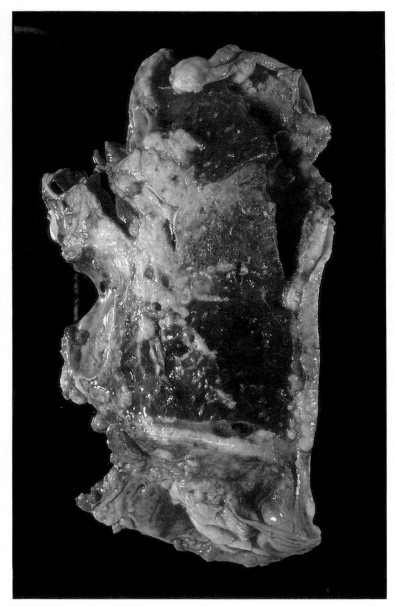

Fig. 3.57

Fig. 3.57 Bronchogenic carcinoma. M/45. The tumour has arisen from the right main bronchus and there are secondaries in the mediastinal lymph nodes and the pleura. In the middle and lower lobes there is tumour spreading along the peribronchial lympatics.

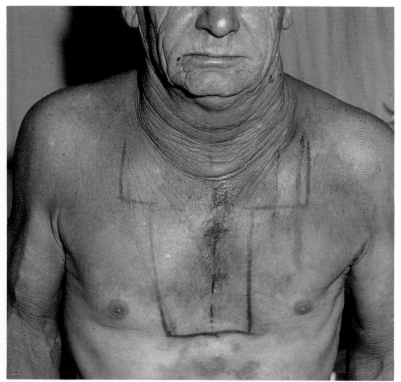

Fig. 3.58

Fig. 3.58 Obstruction of the superior vena cava by a primary lung cancer. M/51. This caused gross swelling of the neck resulting in respiratory obstruction. The patient was having radiotherapy at the time this photograph was taken, but he died a few days later.

Fig. 3.59 Post mortem examination on the patient in Fig. 3.58 shows the lung cancer obstructing the superior vena cava and causing dilatation of the veins draining into it.

Fig. 3.60 Malignant pericarditis. The vascular congestion of the neck was exacerbated by the presence of a secondary tumour in the myocardium and pericardium. Same patient as Fig. 3.58.

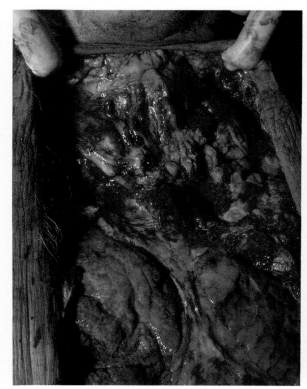

Fig. 3.59

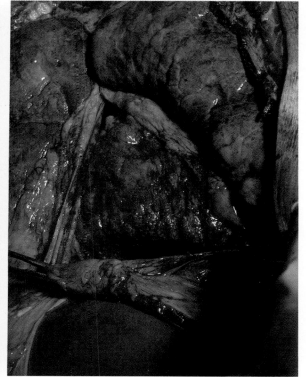

Fig. 3.60

Fig. 3.61 Left-sided pleural mesothelioma. M/50. The left lung is encased in thick, white, hard tumour tissue and there is secondary tumour in the right lung and in the liver. He had been working in an open-cut asbestos mine.

Fig. 3.62 Mesothelioma causing constrictive pericarditis. M/59. The heart has been cut across to show that the pericardial cavity has been completely obliterated by dense, white tissue which was part of a pleural mesothelioma. The patient had worked in an asbestos mine.

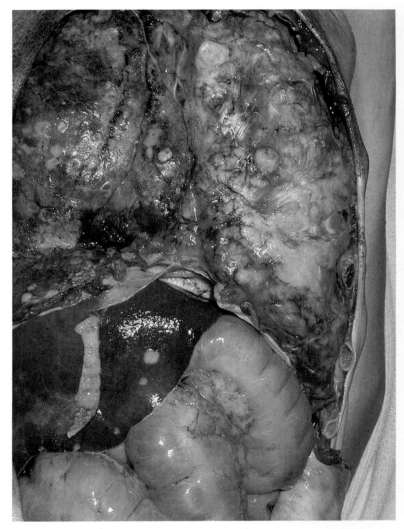

Fig. 3.61

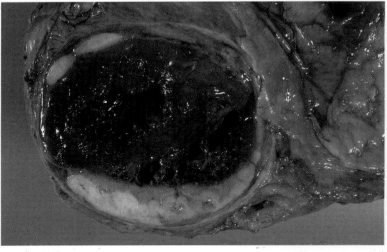

Fig. 3.62

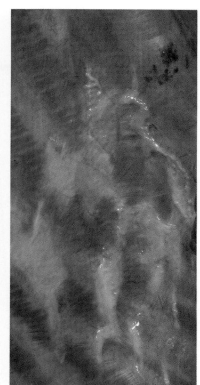

Fig. 3.64

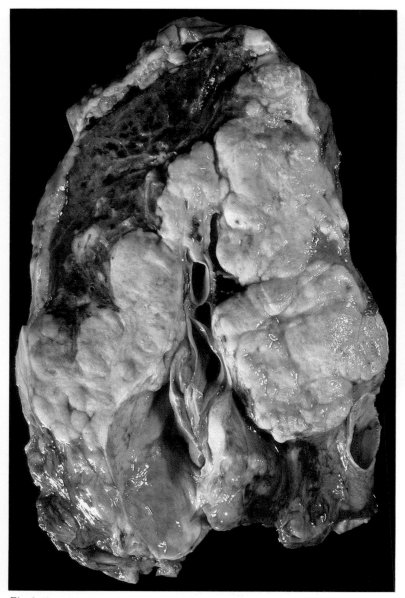

Fig. 3.63

Fig. 3.63 Pleural mesothelioma. M/67. This vertical slice of
the right lung shows the manner in which a pleural
mesothelioma causes thickening of the pleura and encases the
whole lung and the mediastinum.

Fig. 3.64 Pleural plaques. The left parietal pleura of the
patient in Fig. 3.63 showing fibrous plaques running in the line
of the ribs. Pleural plaques indicate previous exposure to
asbestos, but they may occur without causing clinical
symptoms, and without necessarily being associated with any
other manifestation of asbestosis.

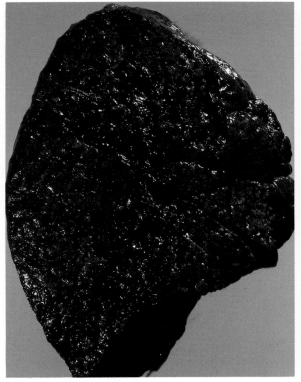

Fig. 3.65

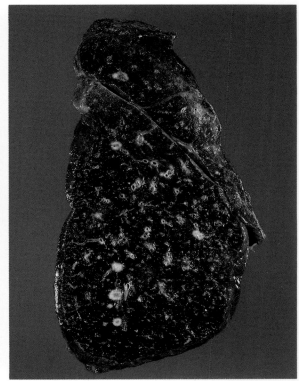

Fig. 3.66

Fig. 3.65 Alveolar cell carcinoma of the lung. F/72. Multiple, rounded, red masses of tumour have developed in all lobes of the lung.

Fig. 3.66 Secondary carcinoma of the lung. F/59. There are a number of rounded nodules of tumour through the lung. The primary was a breast carcinoma.

4

Alimentary system

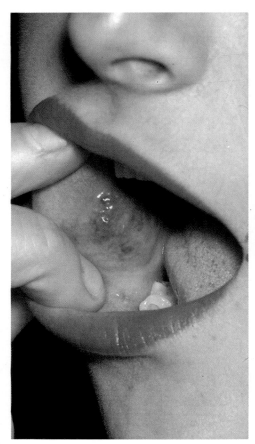

Fig. 4.1

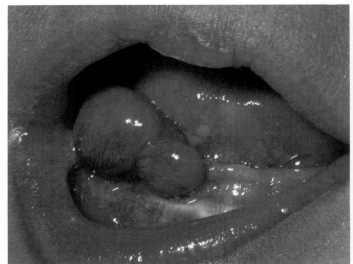

Fig. 4.2

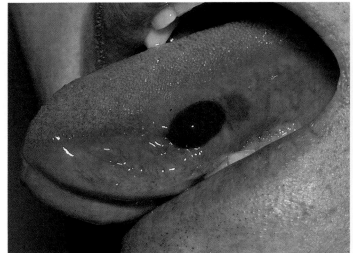

Fig. 4.3

Fig. 4.1 Hemangioma of the buccal mucosa. F/20.

Fig. 4.2 Congenital epulis. F/Neonate. Microscopically this was a granular cell myoblastoma.

Fig. 4.3 Mucus retension cyst of a minor salivary gland on the under surface of the tongue. M/40. This cyst developed within a few hours, persisted for four days, then ruptured.

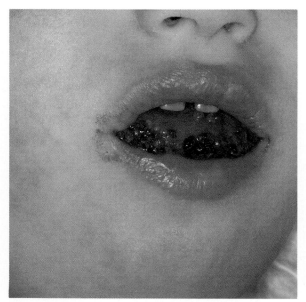

Fig. 4.4

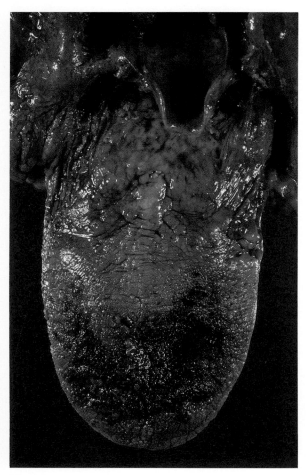

Fig. 4.6

Fig. 4.5

Fig. 4.4 Macroglossia. F/2. This is the normal resting position of her mouth.

Fig. 4.5 Same case as Fig. 4.4. The enlarged tongue has been withdrawn to show the multiple, cystic nodules on its surface. The enlargement was due to the presence of a lymphangioma.

Fig. 4.6 Monilia of the tongue. M/70. The patient died from malignant lymphoma.

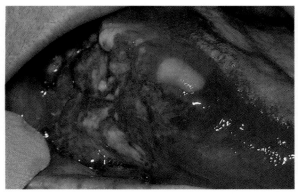

Fig. 4.7

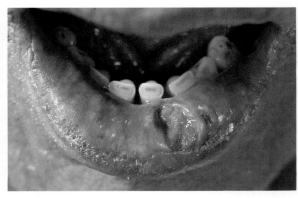

Fig. 4.8

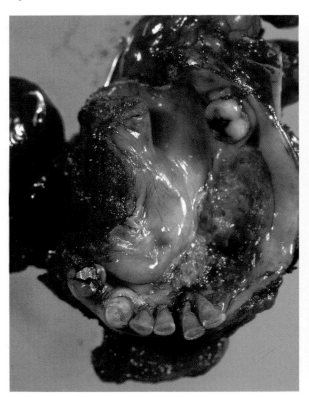

Fig. 4.9

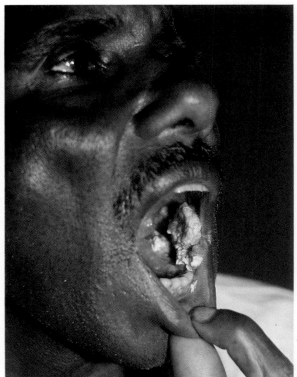

Fig. 4.10

Fig. 4.7 Squamous cell carcinoma of the base of the tongue. F/60.

Fig. 4.8 Squamous cell carcinoma of the lower lip. M/60.

Fig. 4.9 Squamous cell carcinoma of the floor of the mouth. F/77. This cancer was removed surgically and the patient lived for another ten years before dying of an unrelated condition.

Fig. 4.10 Squamous cell carcinoma of the buccal mucosa. Indian M/40 from Bombay. Cancer of this type is very common in all cultures where betel nut is chewed.

Fig. 4.11 Calculus impacted in the duct of a submandibular gland. M/40. Surgically removed to relieve the symptoms of pain and swelling during salivation.

Fig. 4.12 Pleomorphic adenoma of parotid gland. F/52. The multilobulated appearance of this tumour is shown. It must be removed together with some surrounding parotid gland or else some of the irregular projections around its margins will be left behind and the tumour will recur.

Fig. 4.13 Ameloblastoma of maxilla. F/30. A benign, multiloculated neoplasm within the maxilla arising from the enamel organ.

Fig. 4.14 Dentigerous cyst, shelled out from the mandible. M/5. The cyst contains an unerupted tooth.

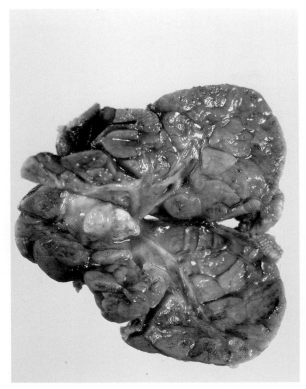

Fig. 4.11

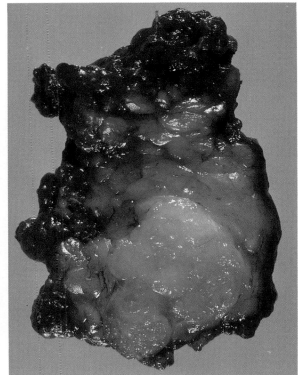

Fig. 4.12

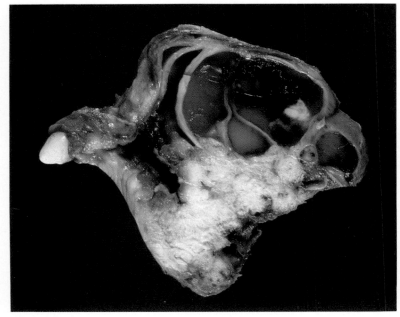

Fig. 4.13

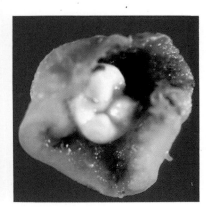

Fig. 4.14

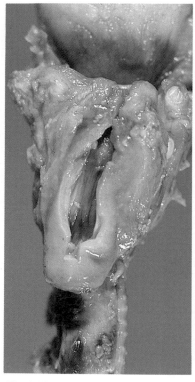

Fig. 4.15

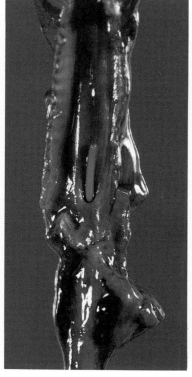

Fig. 4.16

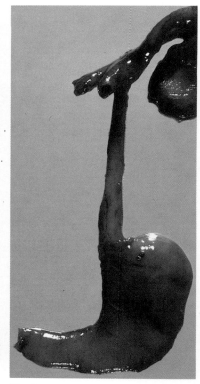

Fig. 4.17

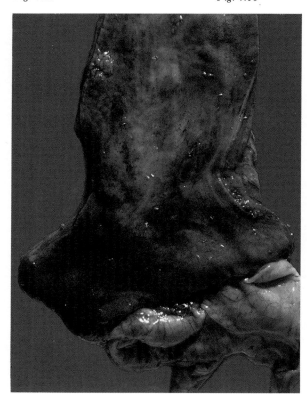

Fig. 4.18

Fig. 4.15 Tracheo-oesophageal fistula. Newborn child. The upper end of the oesophagus terminates as a blind pouch.

Fig. 4.16 The lower half of the abnormality shown in Fig. 4.15. The distal end of the oesophagus opens into the trachea just above the carina.

Fig. 4.17 This shows the entire abnormality with a blindly ending upper oesophageal pouch and the lower part of the oesophagus opening into the trachea proximal to the carina. There are a number of different types of Tracheo-oesophageal fistula. This one is the most common.

Fig. 4.18 Acute on chronic oesophagitis resulting from reflux associated with a hiatus hernia. F/70.

Fig. 4.19 Monilial oesophagitis. M/50. The patient died from malignant lymphoma. The thick, greenish membrane is composed of Candida hyphae and purulent exudate.

Fig. 4.20 Pharyngeal diverticulum. M/73. This was removed surgically to relieve symptoms of dysphagia.

Fig. 4.21 Oesophageal varices. M/70. The patient died from the effects of alcoholic cirrhosis.

Fig. 4.22 Same specimen as Fig. 4.21 transilluminated to accentuate the varices.

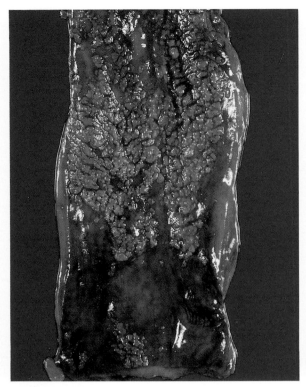

Fig. 4.19

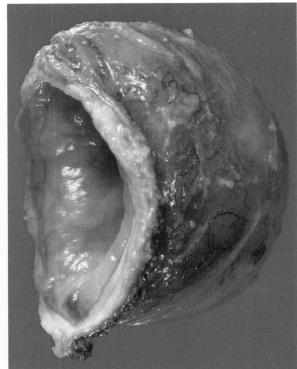

Fig. 4.20

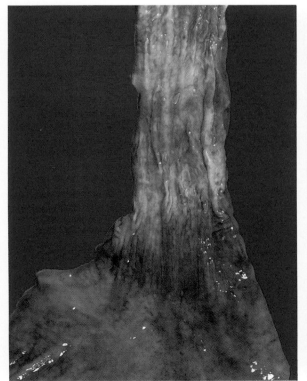

Fig. 4.21

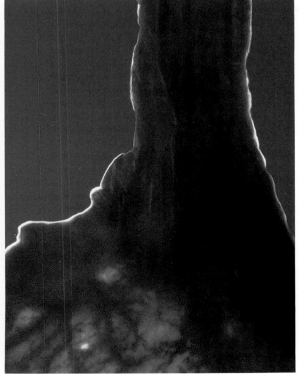

Fig. 4.22

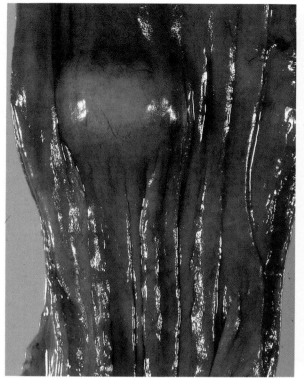

Fig. 4.23

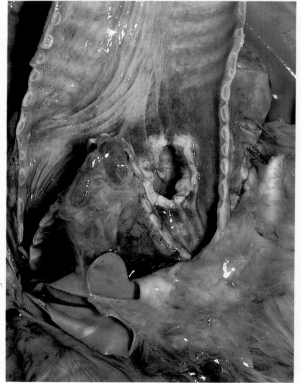

Fig. 4.24

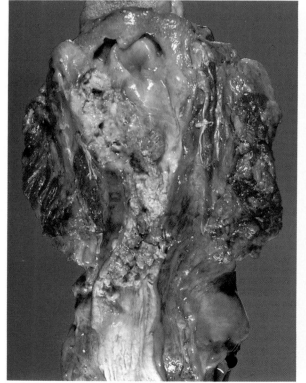

Fig. 4.25

Fig. 4.26

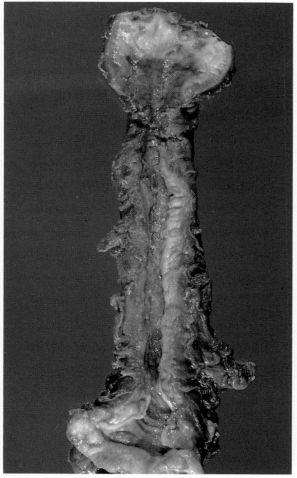

Fig. 4.27

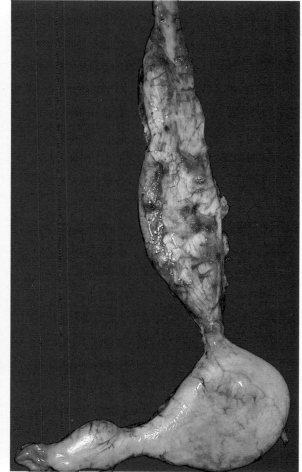

Fig. 4.28

Fig. 4.23 Leiomyoma of the oesophagus. M/51.

Fig. 4.24 Squamous cell carcinoma of the lower third of the oesophagus. M/61.

Fig. 4.25 Squamous cell carcinoma of the upper third of the oesophagus. M/63.

Fig. 4.26 Squamous cell carcinoma of the middle third of the oesophagus eroding into the left main bronchus. M/58.

Fig. 4.27 Oesophageal stricture. F/51. Surgical specimen. The oesophageal wall is fibrotic and the lumen is greatly reduced. This resulted from swallowing caustic soda with suicidal intent.

Fig. 4.28 Megaoesophagus from achalasia of the lower end. M/84. Every day for the 30 years before his death the patient had swallowed a rubber, mercury-filled bougie to dilate the lower end of his oesophagus and relieve his symptoms of dysphagia. He had suffered from a number of episodes of aspiration pneumonia before the one that finally caused his death.

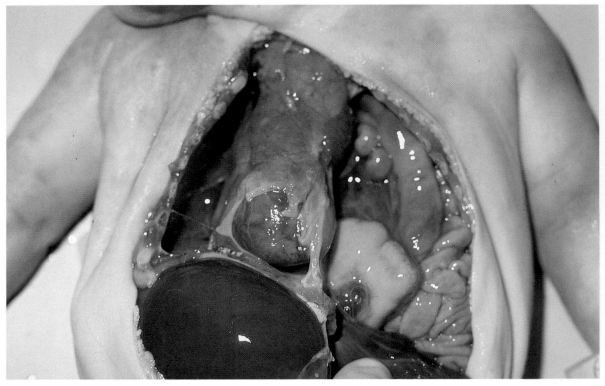

Fig. 4.29

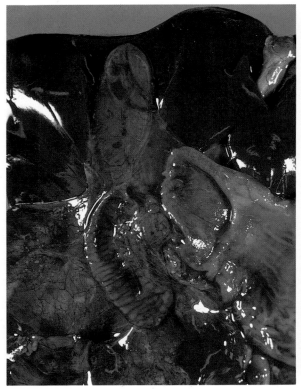

Fig. 4.30

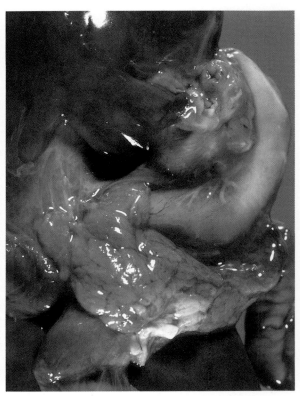

Fig. 4.31

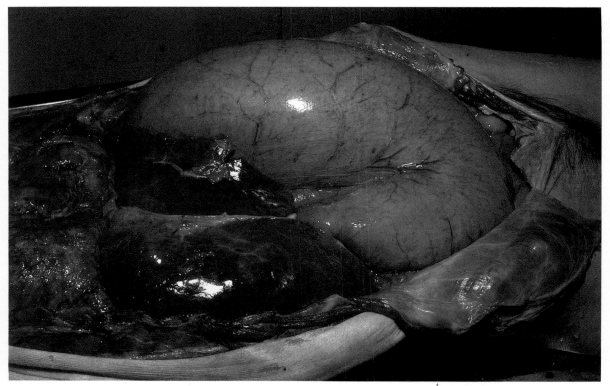

Fig. 4.32

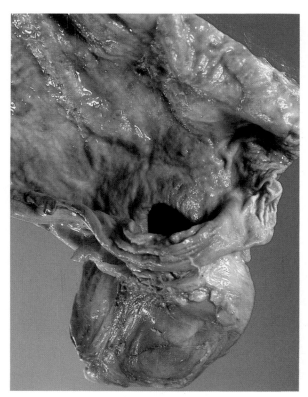

Fig. 4.29 Left-sided congenital diaghragmatic hernia. M/neonate. Abdominal contents are present in the thorax. There is hypoplasia of the left lung and the mediastinum is pushed to the right. Death occurred shortly after delivery.

Fig. 4.30 Duodenal atresia. Neonatal death. The pylorus has been opened and ends blindly. The second part of the duodenum has been opened and it terminates blindly at both ends.

Fig. 4.31 Annular pancreas. M/4 weeks. The head of the pancreas has wrapped around the first and second parts of the duodenum causing pyloric obstruction.

Fig. 4.32 Acute dilatation of the stomach. F/60.

Fig. 4.33 Gastric diverticulum. F/71. Incidental post mortem finding.

Fig. 4.33

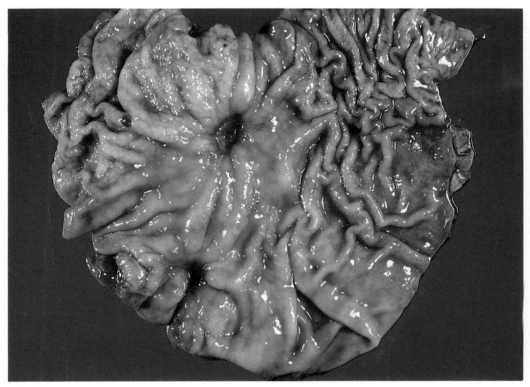

Fig. 4.34

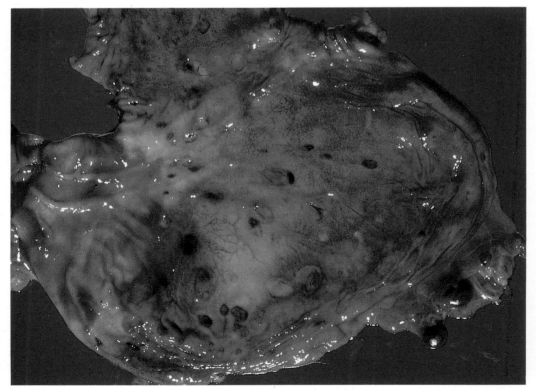

Fig. 4.35

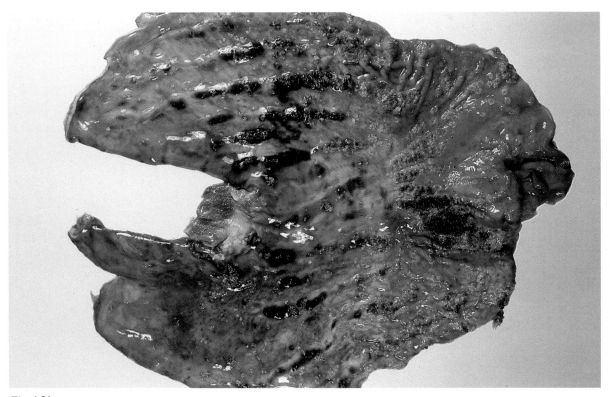

Fig. 4.36

Fig. 4.34 Chronic peptic ulcer. M/44. A partial gastrectomy was performed because of haematemesis. There was a bleeding artery in the base of the ulcer.

Fig. 4.35 Acute gastric erosions. M/78. These occurred just prior to death.

Fig. 4.36 Monilial gastritis. F/11. This child died of aplastic anaemia. The green monilial membrane is adherent to the surfaces of the rugal folds.

Fig. 4.37 Mallory Weiss tear at the oesophago-gastric junction. F/56. The patient died from a massive haematemesis resulting from this tear. A tear in the mucosa at this point characteristically follows an episode of severe vomiting, frequently associated with a bout of heavy drinking.

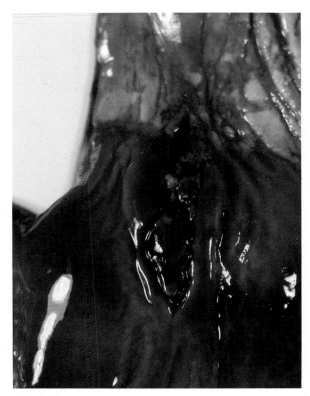

Fig. 4.37

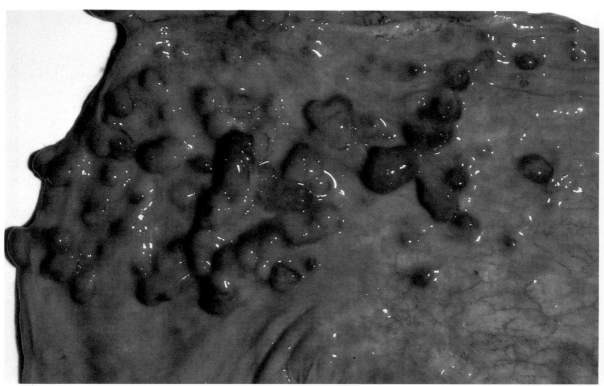

Fig. 4.38

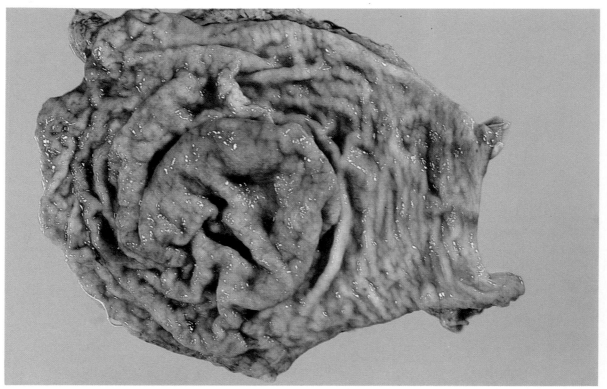

Fig. 4.39

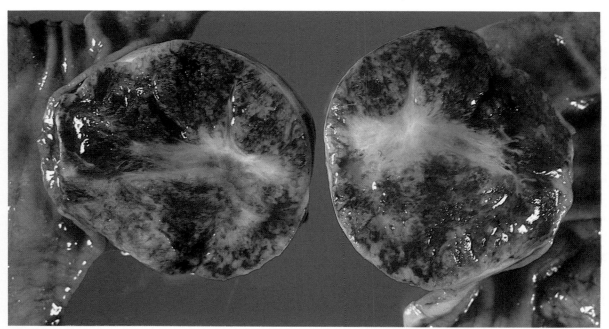

Fig. 4.40

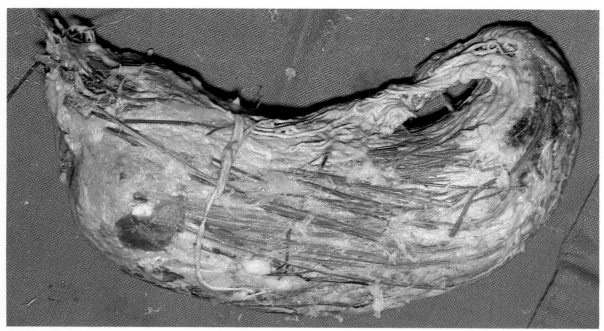

Fig. 4.41

Fig. 4.38 Multiple benign adenomatous gastric polyps. M/75. Incidental post mortem finding.

Fig. 4.39 Giant rugal hypertrophy. M/65. Partial gastrectomy performed because a space occupying lesion was seen on a Barium meal examination and erroneously diagnosed as cancer.

Fig. 4.40 Large leiomyoma of the stomach. F/40. The patient presented with haematemesis from mucosal ulceration on the surface of the tumour.

Fig. 4.41 Bezoir removed from the stomach. M/12. It is composed predominantly of hair and straw. This mentally defective child's usually placid behaviour was replaced by hypermania. Removal of the bezoir restored his placid disposition.

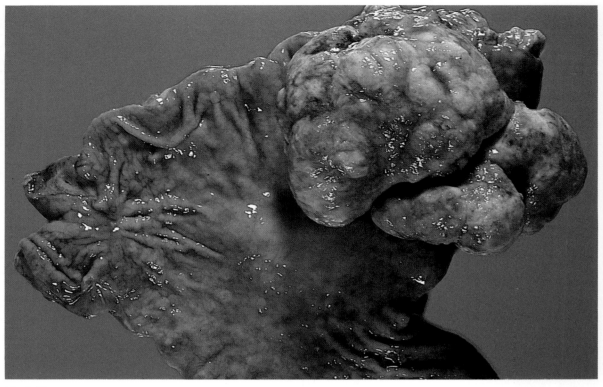

Fig. 4.42

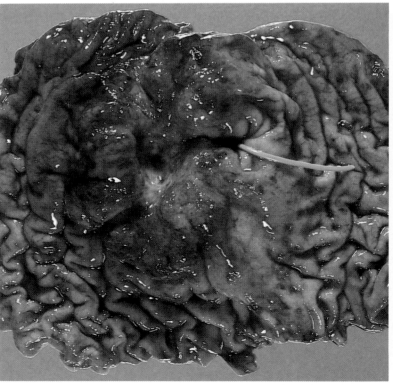

Fig. 4.43

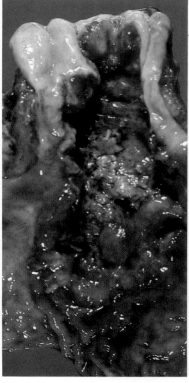

Fig. 4.44

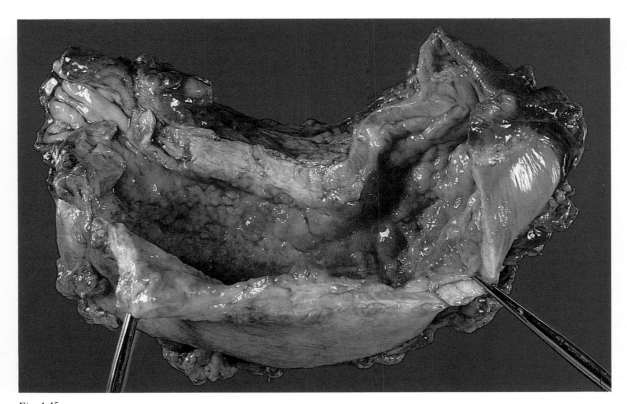

Fig. 4.45

Fig. 4.42 Polypoid adenocarcinoma of stomach. F/86. The
patient was treated by partial gastrectomy.

Fig. 4.43 Ulcerated adenocarcinoma of stomach. M/32. The
patient was treated by partial gastrectomy. The probe is in the
pylorus which was partially obstructed.

Fig. 4.44 Ulcerating adenocarcinoma at the oesophago-gastric
junction. M/50. The tumour was locally resected.

Fig. 4.45 Linitis plastica. F/68. In this type of
adenocarcinoma of the stomach, the tumour cells infiltrate
beneath the mucosa and produce marked fibrosis.

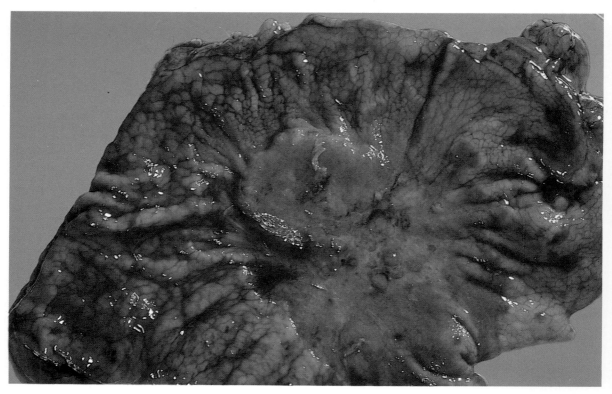

Fig. 4.46

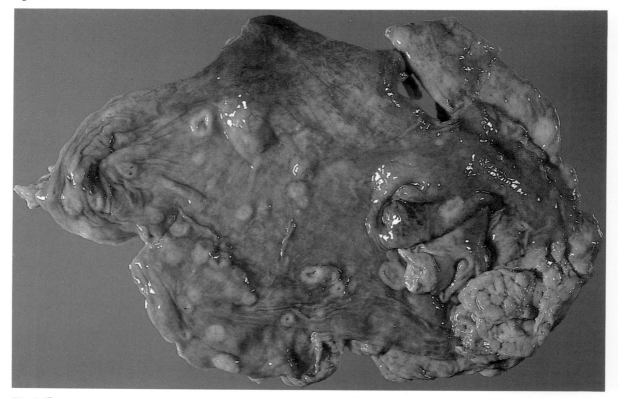

Fig. 4.47

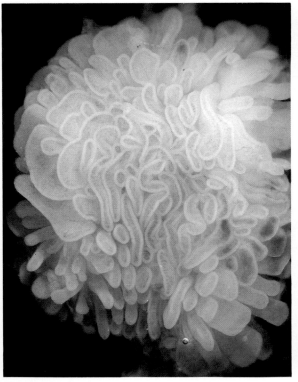

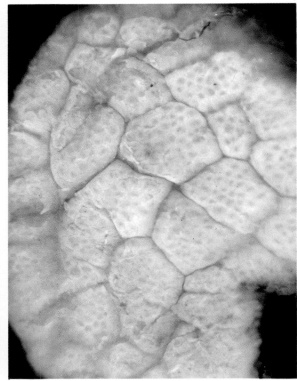

Fig. 4.48   *Fig. 4.49*

Fig. 4.46 Early gastric cancer (superficial adenocarcinoma of the stomach). F/38. The patient was treated by partial gastrectomy. Note the firm, plateau-like area on the stomach mucosa with loss of the rugal folds. The abnormal area in such cases may be better seen by holding the specimen up to the light. This patient had rather vague, non-specific upper abdominal symptoms, and diagnosis was made by gastroscopy and biopsy.

Fig. 4.47 Malignant lymphoma of the stomach. M/60. Note the multiple areas of creamy tumour on the stomach mucosa. The mucosa is ulcerated over some of the deposits.

Fig. 4.48 Normal small intestinal mucosa. F/66. This tissue was obtained by means of a small bowel biopsy capsule and was examined under a dissecting microscope. The intestinal villi appear as fingers, leaves and ridges.

Fig. 4.49 Flat mucosa (total villus atrophy) in coeliac disease. F/31. The patient had had lifelong mild diarrhoea. The jejunal biopsy was performed because her child was diagnosed as having malabsorption syndrome caused by coeliac disease.

Fig. 4.50 Strangulated right inguinal hernia. M/2 months.

Fig. 4.51 The strangulated hernia from Fig. 4.50 was reduced through an incision in the right iliac fossa and the contents were withdrawn from the scrotum. A loop of necrotic bowel can be seen, and this was resected.

Fig. 4.52 Richter's hernia. F/82. In this type of hernia, a portion of the bowel wall slips into the hernial orifice, frequently a femoral hernial orifice, giving rise to intermittent and incomplete intestinal obstruction. This woman died from the effects of complete obstruction when the hernia became impacted in the femoral hernial orifice. The diagnosis was not made during life.

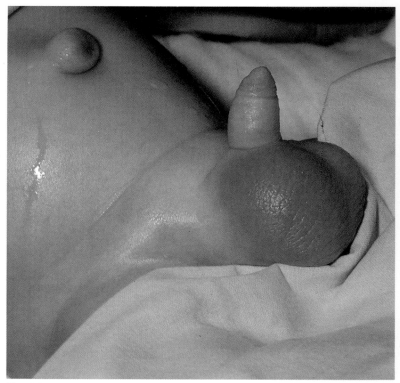

Fig. 4.50

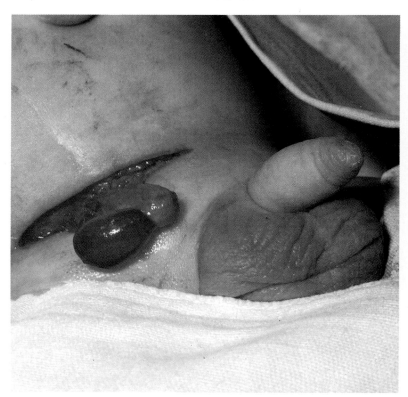

Fig. 4.51

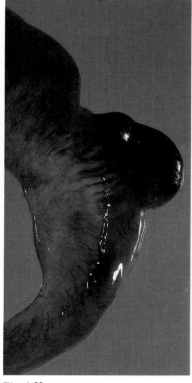

Fig. 4.52

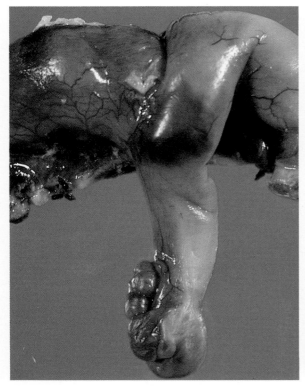

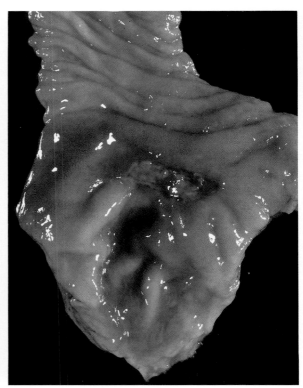

Fig. 4.53

Fig. 4.55

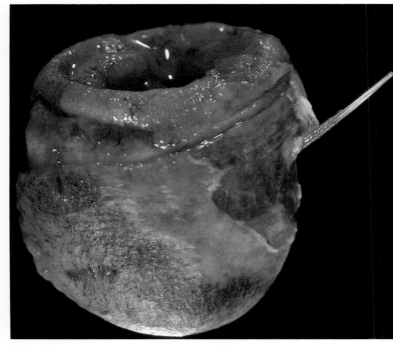

Fig. 4.54

Fig. 4.53 Meckel's diverticulum. M/3 weeks. The Meckel's diverticulum and the adjacent loop of small intestine had become incarcerated in an inguinal hernia and the necrotic bowel segment was resected.

Fig. 4.54 Meckel's diverticulum with a bleeding peptic ulcer.
M/20. This man presented with symptoms and signs of acute appendicitis. At operation the appendix was normal and there was acute inflammation of the Meckel's diverticulum which was perforated by a fish bone, resulting in local peritonitis.

Fig. 4.55 Acute Meckel's diverticulitis. M/25. The ulcer is present at the junction between the diverticulum and the adjoining ileal mucosa at the upper end of the specimen. His presenting symptoms were typical of this condition—sudden onset of abdominal pain closely followed by the passage of bright red blood per rectum.

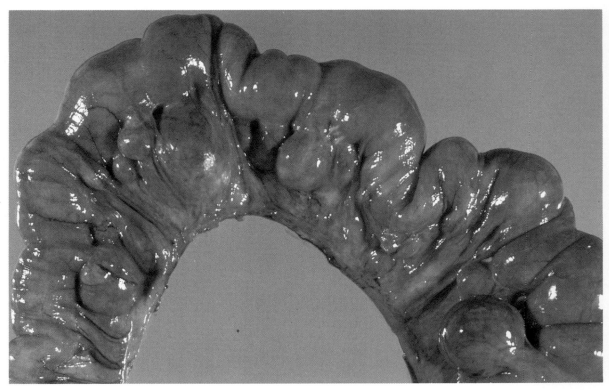

Fig. 4.56

Fig. 4.57

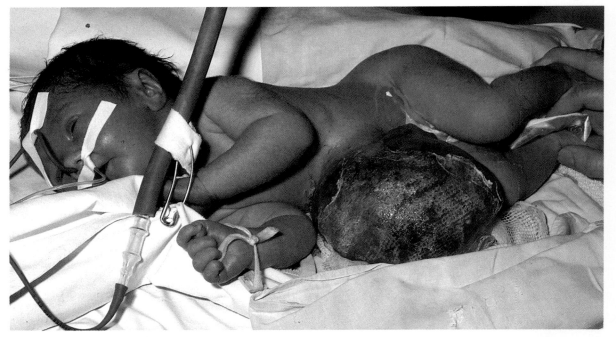

Fig. 4.56 Jejunal diverticula. M/76. An incidental post mortem finding. Note that the diverticula are on the mesenteric border of the bowel, whereas Meckel's diverticulum is on the antimesenteric border.

Fig. 4.57 Exomphalos. M/1 day. There is a defect in the abdominal wall at the umbilicus. The herniated bowel is covered by a thin membrane of amnion. Untreated, death occurs from infection when the membrane ruptures.

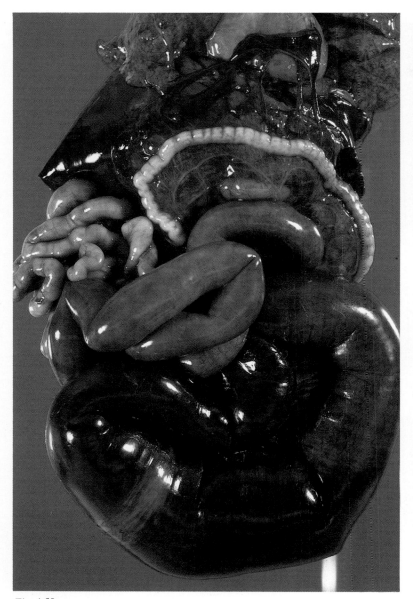

Fig. 4.58

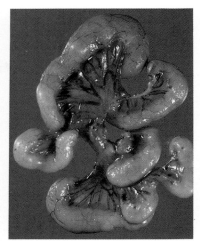

Fig. 4.59

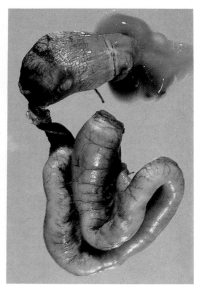

Fig. 4.60

Fig. 4.58 Volvulus of the small intestine. M/2 days. Most of the small intestine is gangrenous, resulting from twisting on its mesentery at the duodeno-jejunal junction.

Fig. 4.59 Multiple areas of atresia in the jejunum. M/2 days. This child presented with intestinal obstruction which was cured by resection of the atretic segment. The atresia consists in multiple, small, blindly-ending segments of intestine.

Fig. 4.60 Meconium ileus. M/6 hours. The neonate presented with intestinal obstruction shortly after delivery. The small intestine is dilated and filled with green, sticky material. This condition represents the presentation of Mucoviscidosis in the neonatal period. The segment of atresia is not related to the Mucoviscidosis.

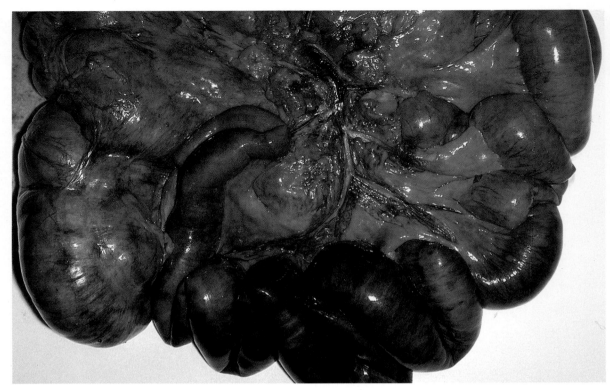

Fig. 4.61

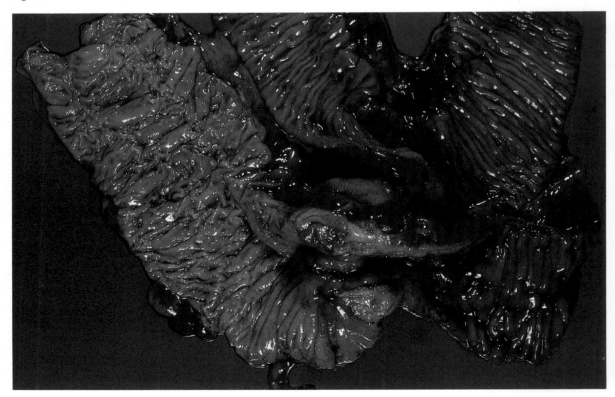

Fig. 4.62

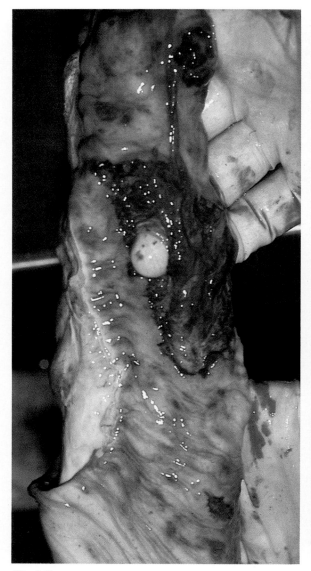

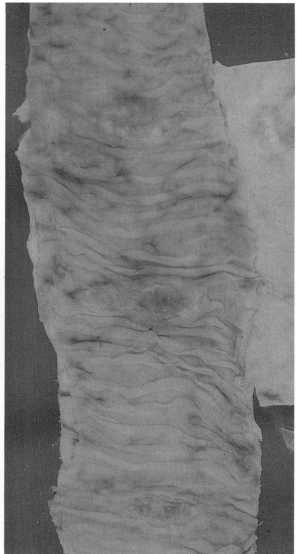

Fig. 4.63

Fig. 4.64

Fig. 4.61 Ischaemic necrosis of the small intestine. F/65.
This was caused by thrombosis of the superior mesenteric
artery displayed in this post mortem specimen.

Fig. 4.62 Crohn's Disease of the terminal ileum. M/21. The
patient presented with recurrent attacks of lower abdominal
pain and vomiting for six weeks. A mass was palpable in the
right iliac fossa. The surgical specimen shows terminal ileum
with a thickened wall and thickening of its mucosal surface—
the so-called 'cobble stone' appearance. An adjacent loop of
ileum has become adherent to it and an ileo-ileal fistula is in the
process of developing.

Fig. 4.63 Typhoid. M/23. Post mortem specimen of small
intestine. The Peyer's patches are prominent. There is
ulceration and haemorrhage into most of them. The
pathologist's finger identifies the site of a perforation in the
middle of the largest area of ulceration and haemorrhage.

Fig. 4.64 Tuberculosis. F/28. Post mortem specimen of small
intestine. There are multiple, oval ulcers running transversely
across the bowel. The patient died from untreated,
disseminated tuberculosis.

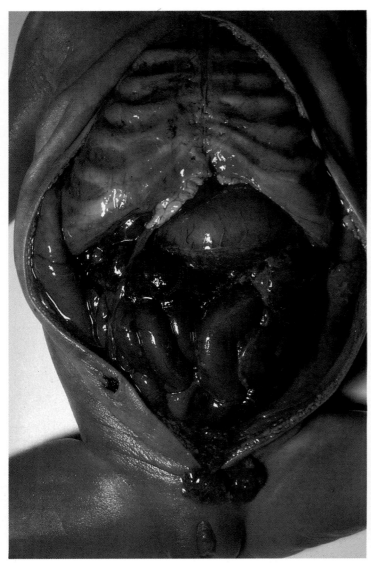

Fig. 4.65

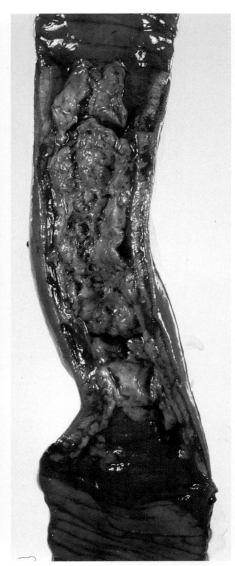

Fig. 4.66

Fig. 4.65 Acute peritonitis resulting from a small perforation in the caecum. Newborn child with **neonatal necrotising enterocolitis**. Note the dilated bowel with a dull red serosal surface on which there is a fibrinous exudate.

Fig. 4.66 Radiation enteritis. M/83. The patient had a carcinoma of the prostate which had been treated by radiotherapy. Some time after this he developed symptoms of intestinal obstruction, and this loop of small intestine which had become incarcerated in the pelvis was resected. The mucosa is ulcerated and lined by a greenish-yellow purulent membrane.

Fig. 4.67 Intussusception causing acute intestinal obstruction. M/33. The apex of the intussusceptum consists of an adenocarcinoma.

Fig. 4.68 Acute obstruction of the ileum. F/80. Examination of the resected bowel showed that the obstruction was caused by a partially dissolved potassium tablet. The bowel is dilated proximal to the obstruction.

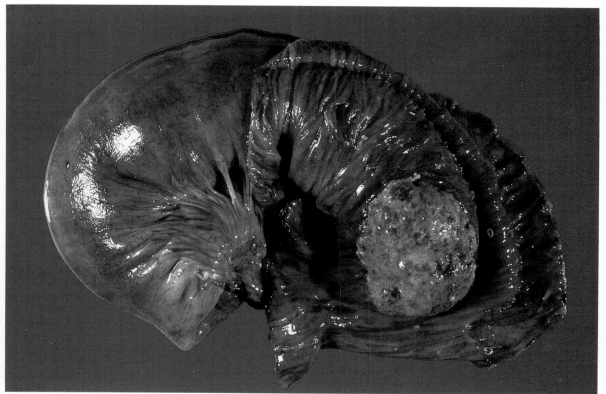

Fig. 4.67

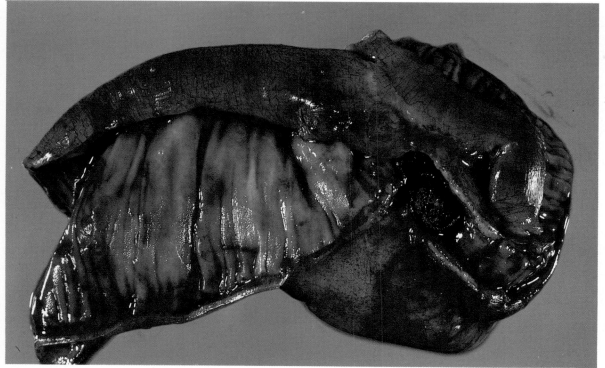

Fig. 4.68

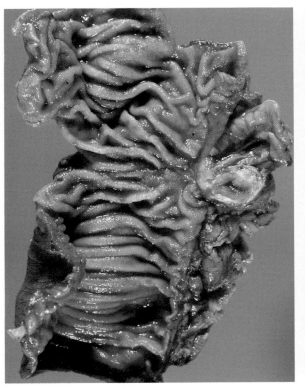

Fig. 4.69

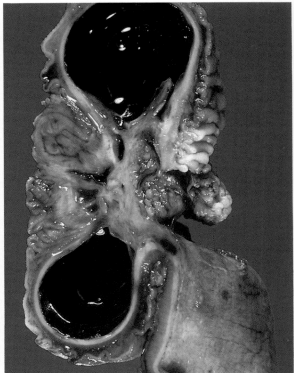

Fig. 4.70

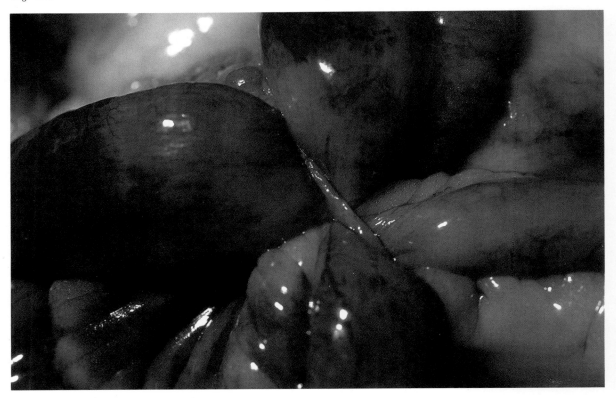

Fig. 4.71

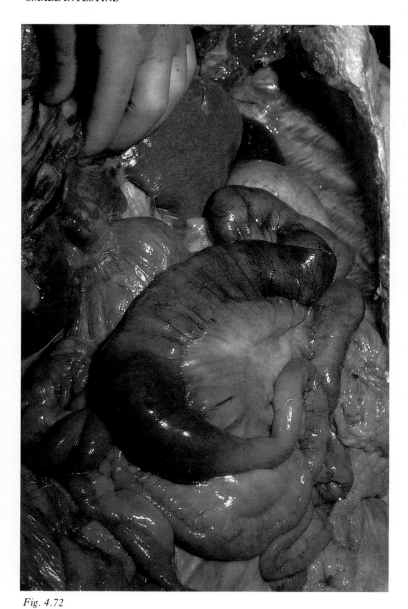

Fig. 4.72

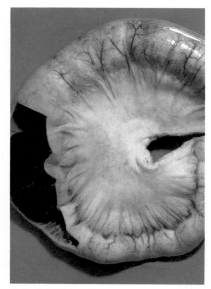

Fig. 4.73

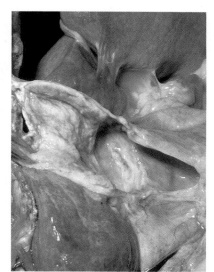

Fig. 4.74

Fig. 4.69 Enterogenous cyst of the ileum. M/48. The small cyst in the ileal wall had caused intestinal obstruction. It consists in a partial duplication of the bowel. Duplications can occur anywhere along the gastrointestinal tract. They are usually short segment duplications and when they cause symptoms, they are those of obstruction.

Fig. 4.70 Endometriosis of the terminal ileum. F/50. This blood-filled cyst had caused intestinal obstruction.

Fig. 4.71 Intestinal obstruction with infarction of a loop of small bowel caused by a fibrous band. M/60. The patient had had an appendicectomy 25 years previously.

Fig. 4.72 Gall stone ileus. F/77. This woman had complained of intermittent abdominal pain for some months. She finally developed complete obstruction, the cause of which was undiagnosed prior to death. There is an obstruction in the small intestine with dilatation proximal to it.

Fig. 4.73 On opening the bowel shown in Fig. 4.72 a large, single gall stone was found.

Fig. 4.74 Same case as Fig. 4.72. A large fistula was present between the gall bladder and the second part of the duodenum. Repeated attacks of cholecystitis resulted in adhesion of the gall bladder to the duodenum. Necrosis of the intervening tissue allowed the gall stone to pass into the duodenum.

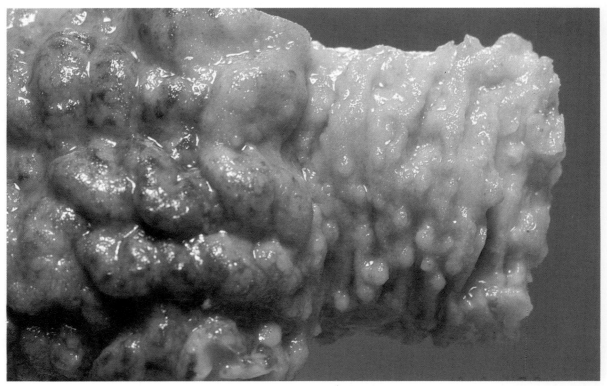

Fig. 4.75

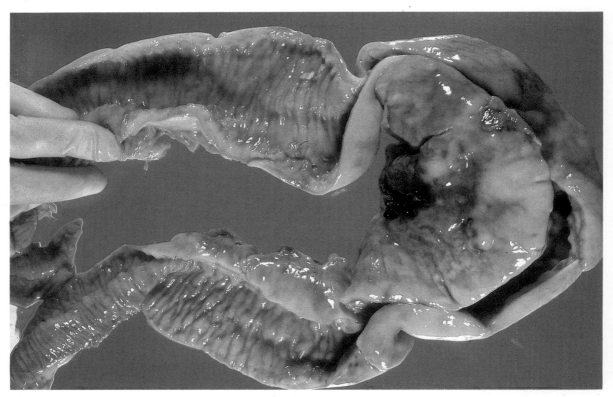

Fig. 4.76

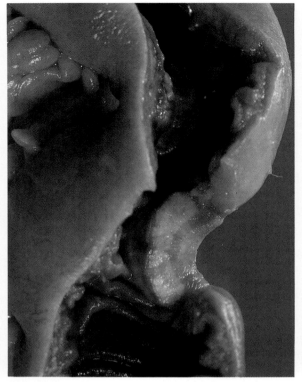

Fig. 4.77

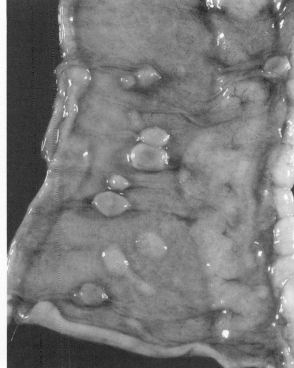

Fig. 4.78

Fig. 4.75 Focal nodular lymphoid hyperplasia of the ileum.
F/9. On the right, small nodules of lymphoid hyperplasia can
be seen. On the left, this hyperplasia has become so gross as to
produce a tumour which resulted in intestinal obstruction
necessitating resection.

Fig. 4.76 Malignant lymphoma of the small intestine. M/3½.
The bowel wall over a long segment has been thickened by a
creamy mass of soft tumour. The mesenteric lymph nodes are
also enlarged.

Fig. 4.77 Carcinoid tumour in the terminal ileum. F/80. The
yellow tumour is protruding into the lumen of the ileum. This
resulted in intestinal obstruction. Such tumours frequently
metastasize to the liver and cause the carcinoid syndrome, but
this patient showed no evidence of that.

Fig. 4.78 Multiple carcinoids in the small intestine. F/61.
Incidental post mortem finding. Carcinoids of the small
intestine are frequently multiple.

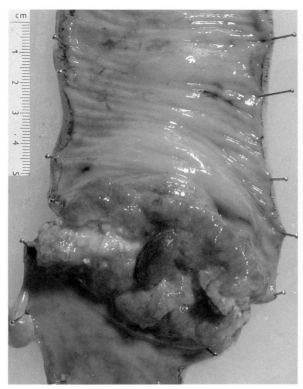

Fig. 4.79

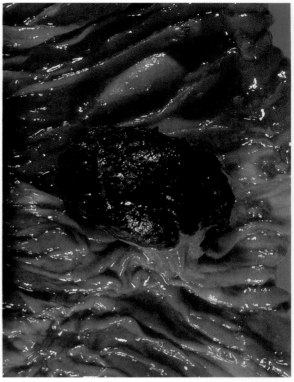

Fig. 4.80

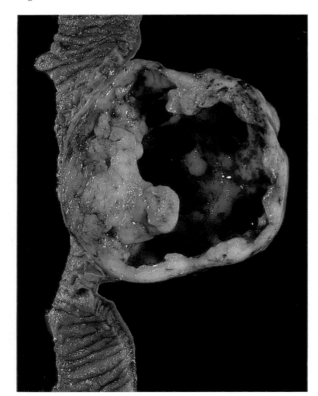

Fig. 4.81

Fig. 4.79 Adenocarcinoma of the ileum. F/63. The patient had had recurrent attacks of abdominal pain and finally came to laparotomy because of acute intestinal obstruction. The obstruction was caused by the lodging of a large fruit seed at the site of partial obstruction caused by the carcinoma. Intestinal obstruction occurs later in small bowel carcinomas than in large bowel carcinomas, because the bowel contents are more liquid in the small intestine.

Fig. 4.80 Secondary melanoma in the small intestine. M/51. This had resulted in intestinal obstruction.

Fig. 4.81 Leiomyosarcoma of the small intestine. M/55. The patient presented with intestinal obstruction. The tumour is large, cystic and partially necrotic.

Fig. 4.82 Acute peritonitis associated with appendicitis. F/18 months. Peritonitis complicates appendicitis more frequently in children than in adults, because in adults the greater omentum is more likely to seal off an acutely inflamed appendix.

Fig. 4.83 Normal appendix.

Fig. 4.84 Acute appendicitis. M/18. The appendix is dilated and its serosal surface is reddened and covered by a fibrino-purulent exudate.

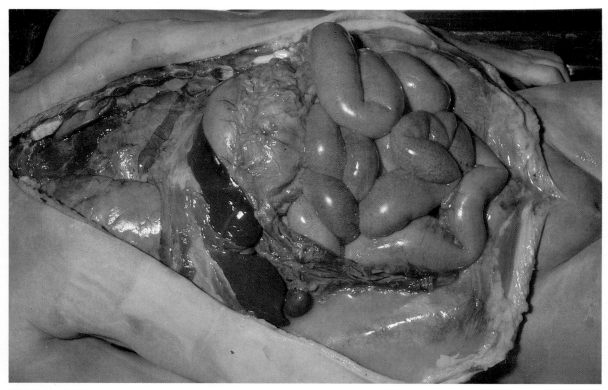

Fig. 4.82

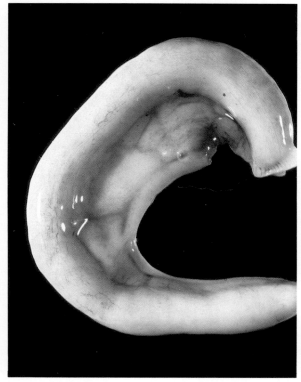

Fig. 4.83

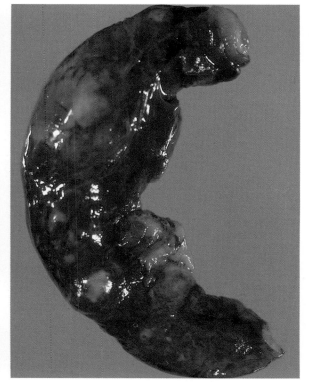

Fig. 4.84

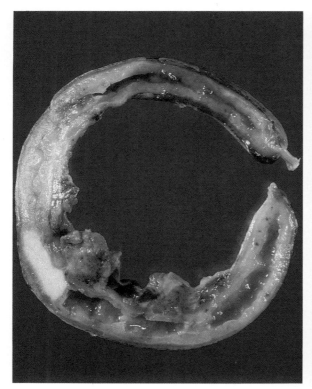

Fig. 4.85

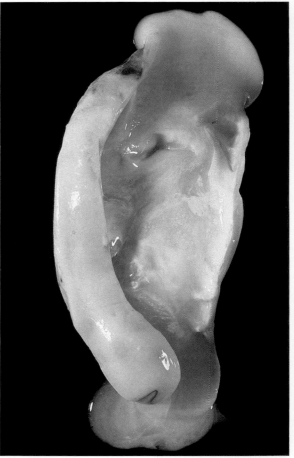

Fig. 4.86

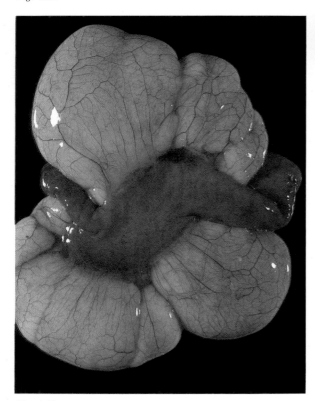

Fig. 4.87

Fig. 4.85 Carcinoid tumour in the appendix. M/24. This was an incidental finding in an appendicectomy for acute appendicitis. The tumour is usually yellow or cream coloured. In this case it is in the middle of the appendix, but it is more often at the tip.

Fig. 4.86 Mucocoele of the appendix. F/40. The appendix is dilated and filled with clear mucus.

Fig. 4.87 Chylous cyst of the mesentery of the small intestine. M/3. The child presented with an abdominal mass.

Fig. 4.88 Acquired megacolon. M/23. The patient was mentally retarded and living in an institution. The megacolon was not related to the cause of death.

Fig. 4.89 Hirschprung's Disease. M/1 week. The baby had been constipated since birth and showing signs of intestinal obstruction. Barium enema showed a narrowed lower rectal segment with dilated rectum above it. This operative photograph shows the typical appearance of Hirschprung's Disease. There are no ganglion cells in the narrowed segment. The lower suture is at the site of biopsy of the intermediate zone in which there are no ganglion cells but nerve fibres between the two muscle layers of the bowel wall. There are normal ganglion cells in the dilated segment—the 'cone'.

Fig. 4.90 Imperforate anus. M/Newborn.

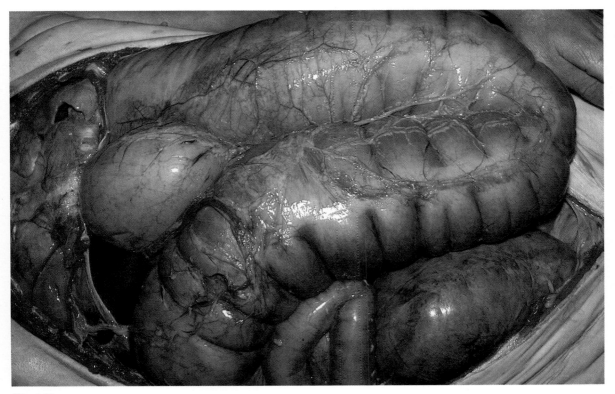

Fig. 4.88

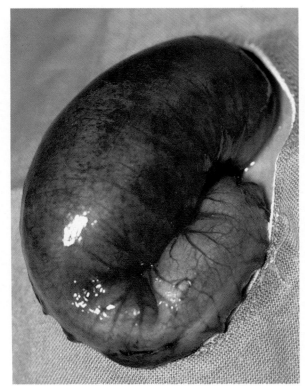

Fig. 4.89

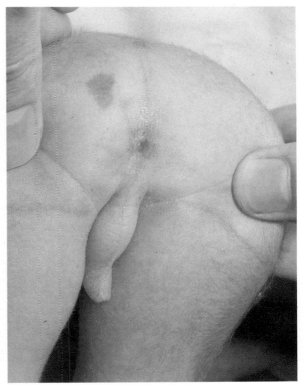

Fig. 4.90

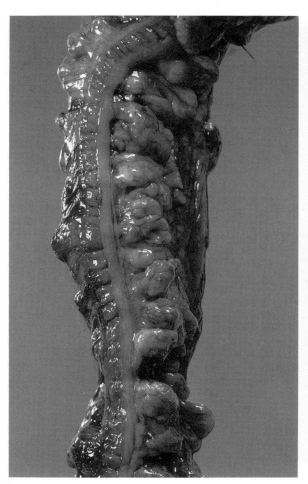

Fig. 4.91

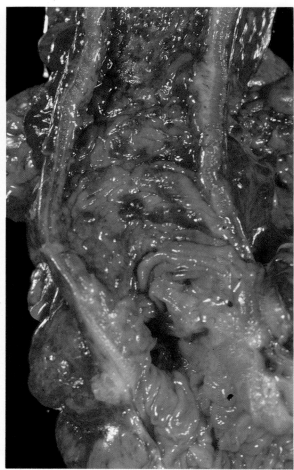

Fig. 4.92

Fig. 4.91 Diverticulosis of the sigmoid colon. F/59. An incidental post mortem finding.

Fig. 4.92 Chronic diverticulitis. F/75. A resected segment of thickened, fibrotic sigmoid colon that had caused obstruction. There is acute colitis proximal to the obstruction.

Fig. 4.93 Melanosis coli. F/73. Note the black colouration of the mucosa throughout the whole length of the colon, whereas the terminal ileum is a normal colour.

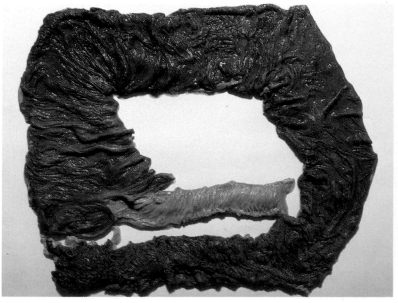

Fig. 4.93

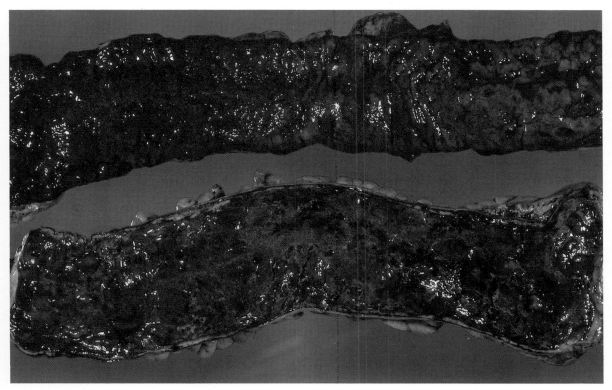

Fig. 4.94

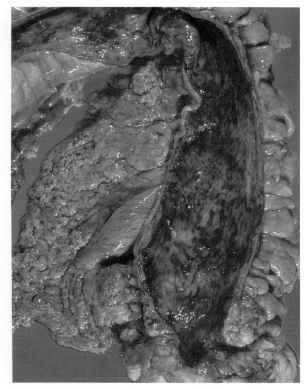

Fig. 4.95

Fig. 4.94 Acute ulcerative colitis. F/16. The mucosa throughout the length of the colon is reddened, oedematous, ulcerated and bleeding. Colectomy was performed because the patient was not responding to medical treatment.

Fig. 4.95 Chronic ulcerative colitis. F/58. The bowel is shortened and its wall is fibrotic. The mucosa is reddened and atrophic. The disease had been present for over 10 years and colectomy was performed, partly to relieve symptoms of diarrhoea and partly to prevent the development of cancer.

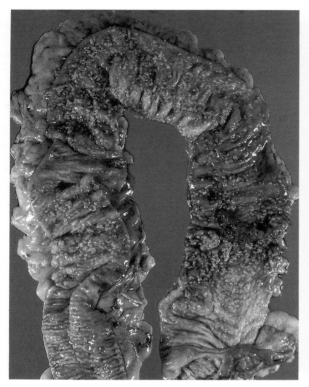

Fig. 4.96

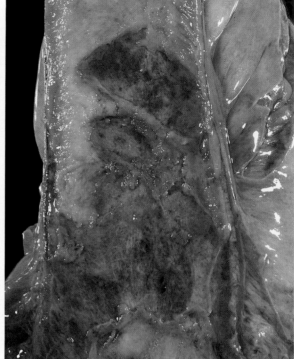

Fig. 4.97

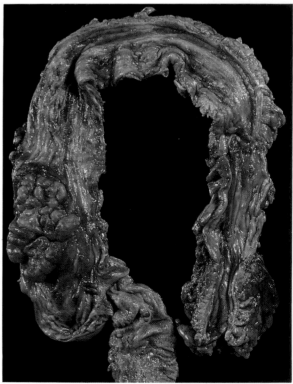

Fig. 4.96 Chronic ulcerative colitis with hyperplastic polyps.
F/40. Colectomy was performed because of longstanding
disease. Virtually the whole of the mucosal surface has been
converted into polyps which have resulted from re-
epithelialisation after the initial ulceration.

Fig. 4.97 Chronic ulcerative colitis with mucosal dysplasia in
the sigmoid colon. F/49. The abnormal areas were seen during
routine colonoscopy to assess the progress of the disease.
Biopsy showed severe dysplasia and colectomy was performed
to prevent the development of carcinoma.

Fig. 4.98 Chronic ulcerative colitis with a carcinoma arising in
the caecum. F/30. An ileo-colectomy was performed. The
patient had had longstanding ulcerative colitis and the
carcinoma was found on colonoscopy.

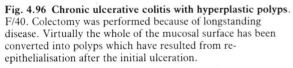

Fig. 4.98

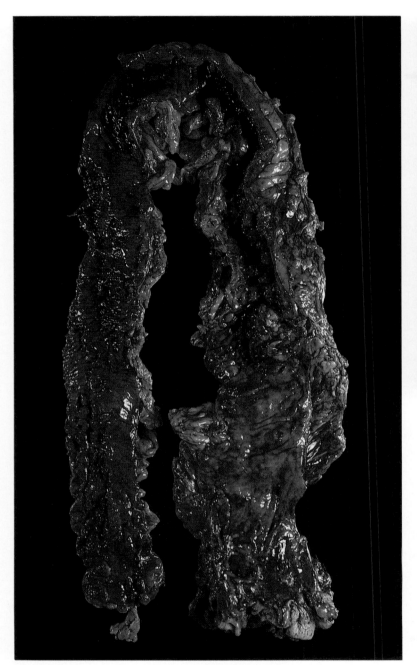

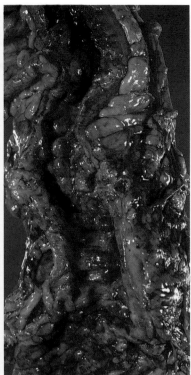

Fig. 4.100

Fig. 4.99

Fig. 4.99 Crohn's Disease of the colon. F/60. Total colectomy performed for disease which could not be controlled by medical treatment. Nearly the whole length of the colon is involved; but there is a segment in the sigmoid colon that is less involved than the rest. In advanced cases such as this it is not easy to identify the segmental involvement characteristic of Crohn's Disease of the colon.

Fig. 4.100 Closer view of the splenic flexure of the specimen in Fig. 4.99 showing thickening of the wall and a 'cobble stone' appearance of the mucosal surface.

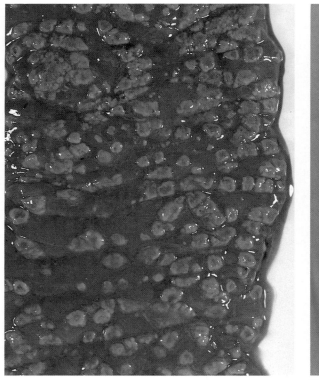

Fig. 4.101

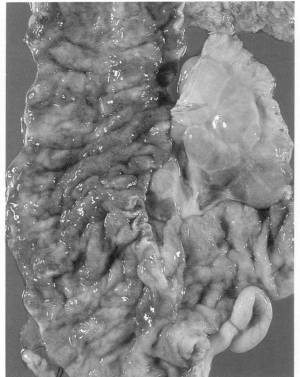

Fig. 4.102

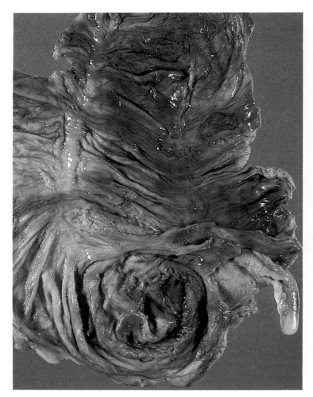

Fig. 4.103

Fig. 4.104

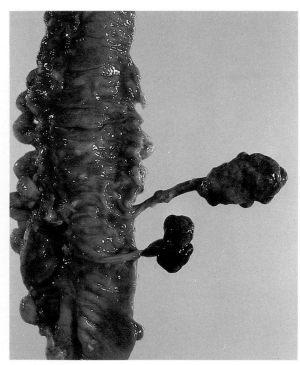

Fig. 4.105

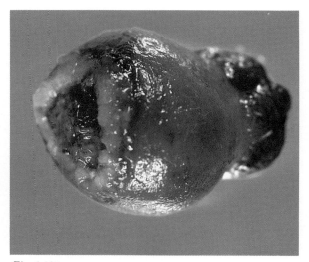

Fig. 4.106

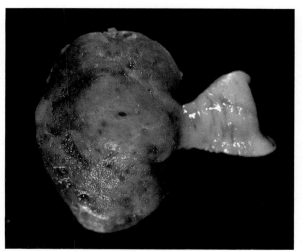

Fig. 4.107

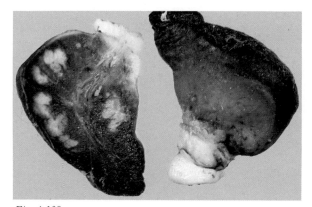

Fig. 4.108

Fig. 4.101 Pseudomembranous colitis. F/68. Colectomy was performed because the patient developed toxic megacolon. She was taking ampicillin and this allowed overgrowth of the Clostridium difficile which produced the multiple, discrete, white plaques of purulent exudate on the mucosal surface.

Fig. 4.102 Ischaemic colitis. M/64. Surgical resection of the splenic flexure following abdominal pain and diarrhoea. The mucosal surface is reddened and covered by a fibrino-purulent exudate. The colon adjacent to this area appears normal.

Fig. 4.103 Amoebic colitis. M/49. Multiple, undermined mucosal ulcers can be seen in the caecum and ascending colon. This man had colitis and liver abscess. While undergoing treatment he suddenly developed an acute pericardial effusion and died.

Fig. 4.104 Acute enterocolitis caused by Shigella. F/19 months. A Shigella organism was isolated from the faeces prior to death. The mucosal surface is reddened and slightly thickened. This infection results in a less florid macroscopic appearance than is seen in the other forms of colitis.

Fig. 4.105 Benign tubular adenomatous polyps of the colon. M/46. These were asymptomatic.

Fig. 4.106 Tubular adenoma removed via a colonoscope. M/73. This polyp was causing rectal bleeding from the ulcer on its surface.

Fig. 4.107 Juvenile polyp. F/7½. This was removed via a colonoscope. These polyps are characterised by the presence of greatly dilated mucus glands which can be seen on its surface.

Fig. 4.108 Hamartomatous polyp from the rectum. M/6 weeks. This had caused rectal bleeding. It is composed of vascular, fibro fatty tissue.

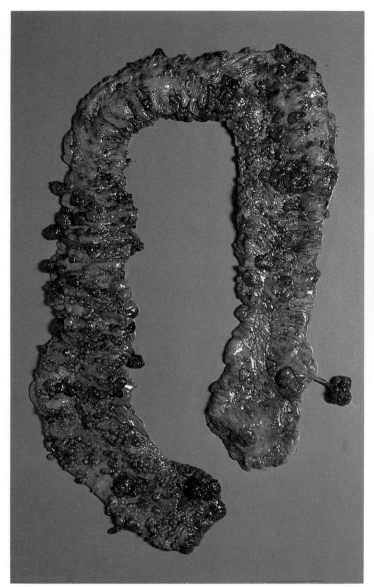

Fig. 4.109

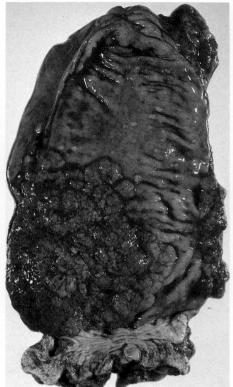

Fig. 4.110

Fig. 4.109 Multiple polyposis coli. F/25. This patient's father had been treated for carcinoma of the colon, and colectomy was performed because of the high risk of her developing a carcinoma. Polyps cover virtually the whole of the mucosal surface of the colon.

Fig. 4.110 Villous papilloma of the rectum. F/48. These polyps are sessile, soft on palpation, and cover quite a large area. They carry a high risk of developing carcinoma.

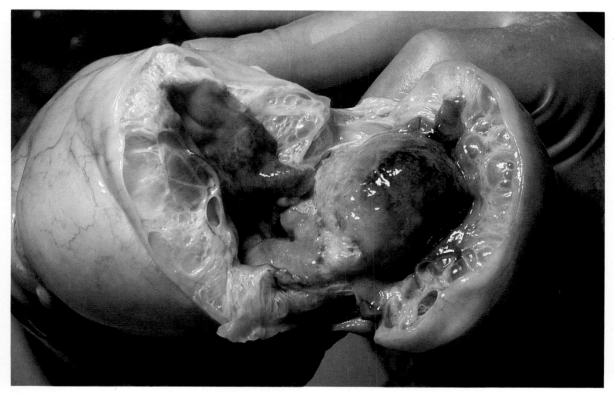

Fig. 4.111

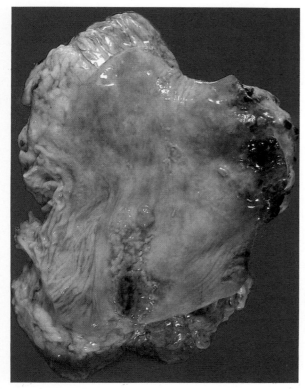

Fig. 4.112

Fig. 4.111 Pneumatosis intestinalis. M/70. The gas-filled cysts caused marked thickening of the colonic wall. This condition can be found in both small and large intestine, but it is most often seen in the colon, where it usually involves a short segment only. This man had the whole length of his colon involved and it was an incidental post mortem finding.

Fig. 4.112 Solitary ulcer of the rectum. M/48. Local resection was performed because of recurrent pain and bleeding.

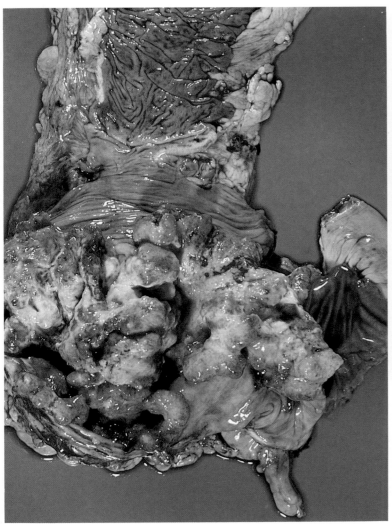

Fig. 4.113

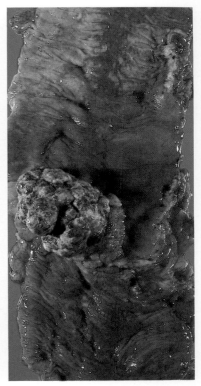

Fig. 4.114

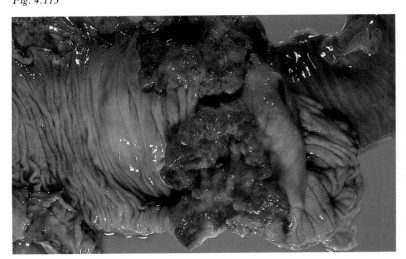

Fig. 4.115

Fig. 4.113 Adenocarcinoma of the caecum. M/53. This tumour is large and its surface is ulcerated and bleeding. These tumours often present in an advanced stage, and frequently because of symptoms of iron deficiency anaemia resulting from chronic blood loss.

Fig. 4.114 Polypoid adenocarcinoma of the colon. M/26. When a carcinoma appears at this young age, it is necessary to exclude the presence of some premalignant condition, for example, polyposis coli. There was no such history in this man.

Fig. 4.115 Adenocarcinoma of the transverse colon. F/87. This tumour is partly polypoid but it had encircled the bowel wall and caused obstruction.

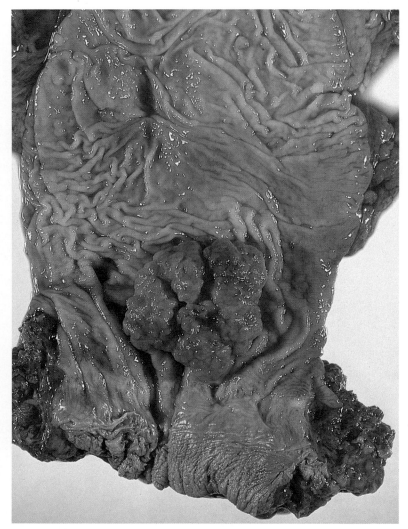

Fig. 4.116

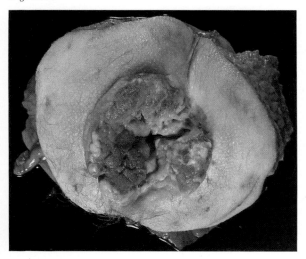

Fig. 4.117

Fig. 4.116 Adenocarcinoma of the rectum. M/70. These tumours frequently present at an early stage in their development with rectal bleeding.

Fig. 4.117 Squamous cell carcinoma of the anus. M/62.

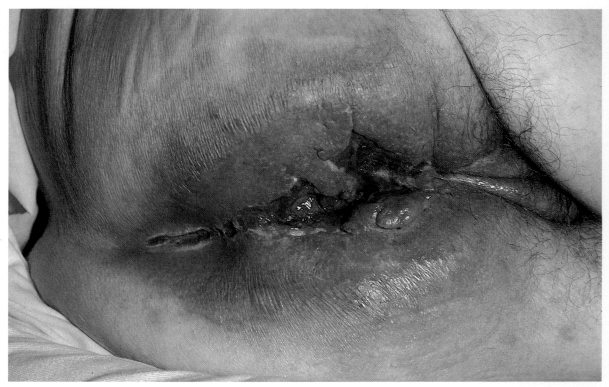

Fig. 4.118

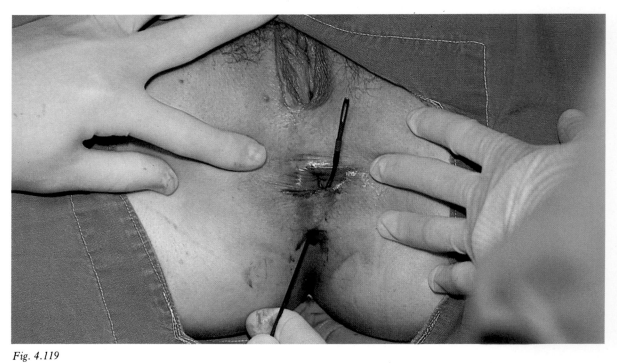

Fig. 4.119

Fig. 4.118 Perianal abscesses and fistulae. F/72. This
complicated her longstanding Crohn's Disease of the colon.

Fig. 4.119 Simple fistula in ano. F/40.

5

Pancreas, biliary system and liver

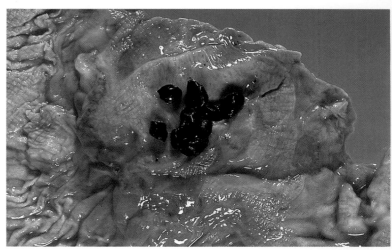

Fig. 5.1

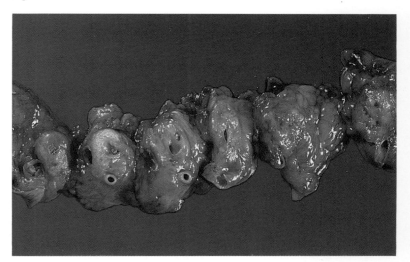

Fig. 5.2

Fig. 5.1 Calculi in the ampulla of Vater.
F/87. There are multiple calculi impacted
in the ampulla. The duodenal surface on
the left is ulcerated as a result of a failed
endoscopic attempt to remove them prior
to death from liver failure.

**Fig. 5.2 Pancreatic atrophy caused by
obstruction of the pancreatic duct by a
calculus**. M/44. The pancreas has been
sliced along its length. The pancreatic
duct in the middle of the gland is dilated,
and there is atrophy of the acinar tissue.
This was an incidental finding in a patient
who died from a carcinoma of the
pharynx.

**Fig. 5.3 Nodule of ectopic pancreas on
the surface of the jejunum**. F/69. An
incidental post mortem finding. Ectopic
pancreatic tissue is found especially in the
pylorus, duodenum and jejunum.

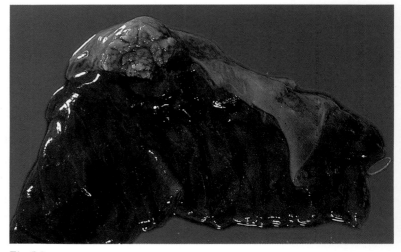

Fig. 5.3

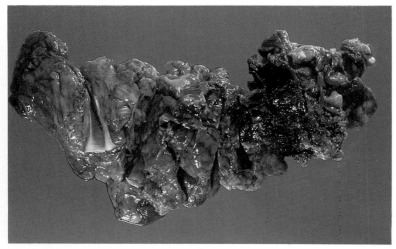

Fig. 5.4

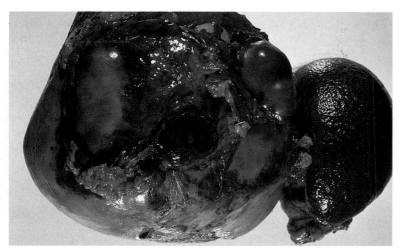

Fig. 5.5

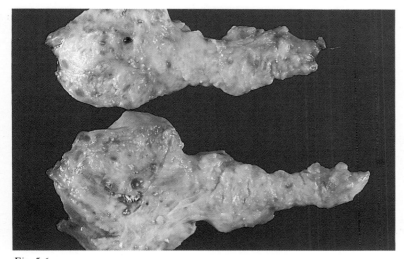

Fig. 5.6

Fig. 5.4 Acute haemorrhagic pancreatitis. M/44. This was the cause of death. Note the haemorrhage, necrosis and yellow spots of enzymatic fat necrosis.

Fig. 5.5 Pseudocyst in the body and tail of the pancreas. F/67. This is a well-recognised complication of acute pancreatitis.

Fig. 5.6 Chronic pancreatitis. F/43. The pancreas is atrophic and fibrotic. The main pancreatic duct is dilated and there are calculi in the ducts in the head of the pancreas. The patient was an alcoholic.

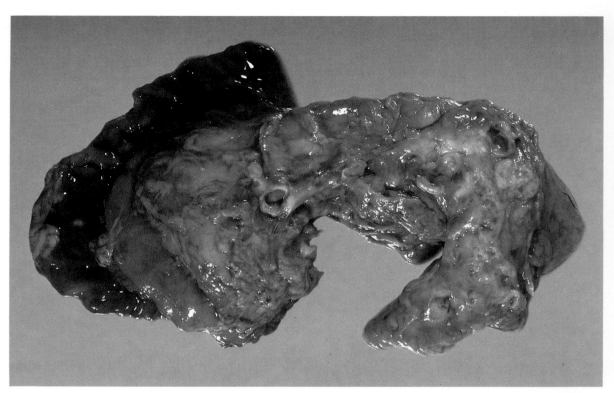

Fig. 5.7

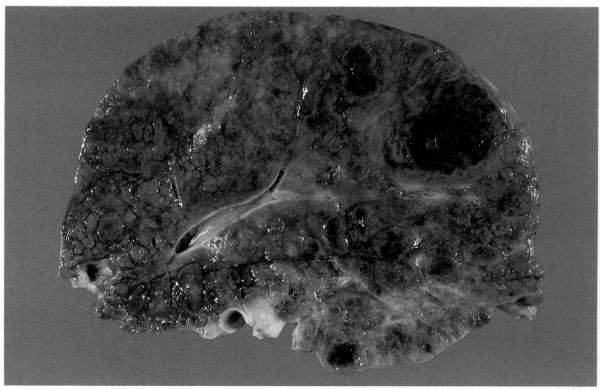

Fig. 5.8

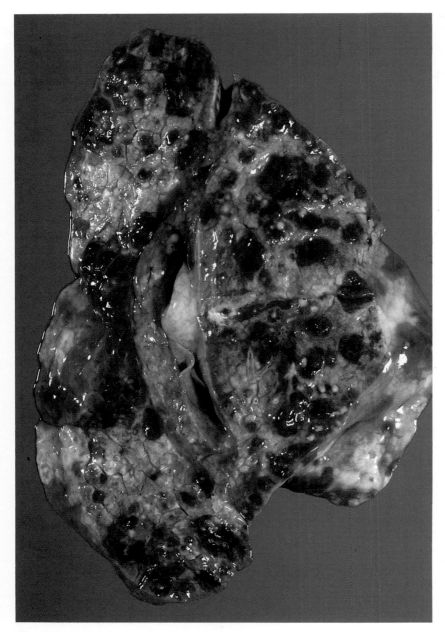

Fig. 5.9

**Fig. 5.7 Fibrocystic disease of the pancreas
(mucoviscidosis).** M/11. The pancreas is viewed from its
posterior surface. The normal tissue is almost completely
replaced by cysts in a fibrotic stroma.

Fig. 5.8 Hepatic cirrhosis in mucoviscidosis. M/6. Cirrhosis
complicates mucoviscidosis in a proportion of cases, usually
presenting about this age as haematemesis.

Fig. 5.9 Lung from a patient with mucoviscidosis. F/2. The
lung shows widespread bronchpneumonia with pus issuing
from dilated bronchi and bronchioles. Recurrent respiratory
tract infection is one of the main complications of this disease.

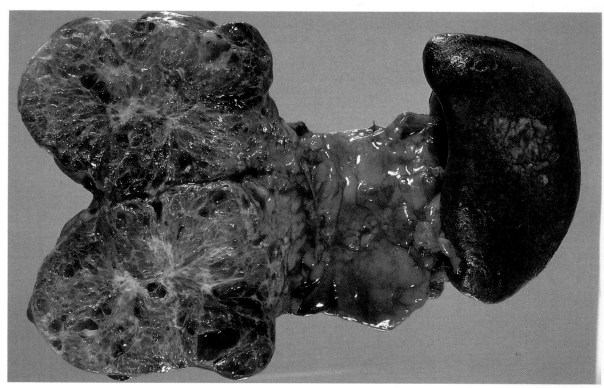

Fig. 5.10

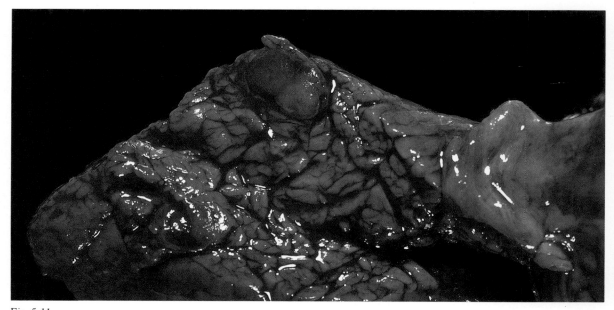

Fig. 5.11

Fig. 5.10 Benign cystadenoma of the head of the pancreas. F/74. The patient presented with an epigastric mass.

Fig. 5.11 Insulin secreting islet cell adenoma of the pancreas. F/45. For many years the patient had had difficulty in waking in the morning, using an alarm clock for this purpose. After a cup of tea with milk and sugar she would feel better and ready for the day. This ultimately became such a problem that she sought medical advice. The diagnosis was made and the adenoma was successfully removed.

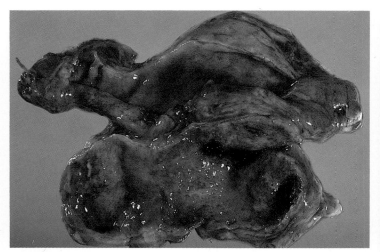

Fig. 5.12

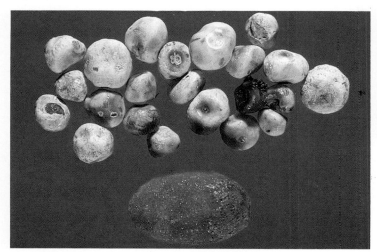

Fig. 5.13

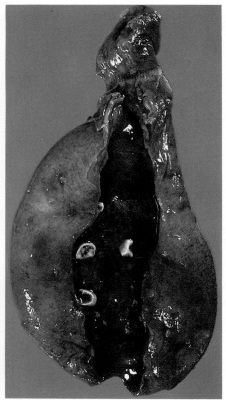

Fig. 5.14

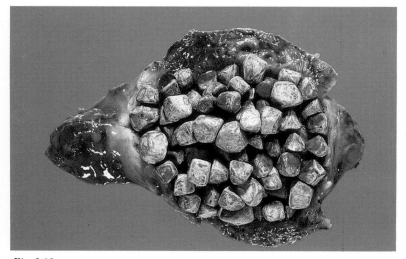

Fig. 5.15

Fig. 5.12 Double gall bladder. F/45. This congenital abnormality was discovered when cholecystectomy was being performed for chronic calculous cholecystitis.

Fig. 5.13 Calculi removed from the gall bladder in Fig. 5.12. One gall bladder contained a single large calculus and the other contained multiple calculi.

Fig. 5.14 Acute on chronic cholecystitis. F/38. The gall bladder is distended. Both serosal and mucosal surfaces are reddened and inflamed. The wall of the gall bladder is thickened and there are a few mixed calculi within it.

Fig. 5.15 Chronic cholecystitis. F/48. The gall bladder shows the features of chronic cholecystitis and it is packed with small multifaceted mixed gall stones.

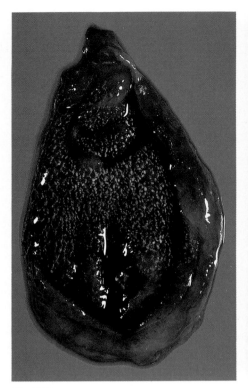

Fig. 5.16

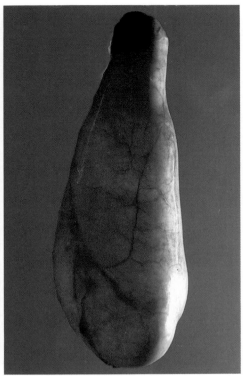

Fig. 5.17

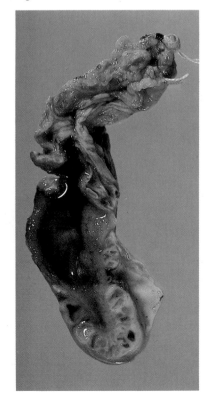

Fig. 5.18

Fig. 5.16 Cholesterolosis. F/36. The gall bladder shows chronic cholecystitis. There are multiple yellow spots on its mucosal surface. This is due to the accumulation of lipid in the lamina propria.

Fig. 5.17 Mucocoele of the gall bladder. M/38. The unopened gall bladder has been transilluminated to show that its wall is thin and it contains semitransparent fluid.

Fig. 5.18 Adenomyoma of the gall bladder. F/50. There is a cream coloured thickening of the fundus at the lower end of the specimen. As is usual, the gall bladder was removed for symptoms of chronic cholecystitis and the presence of the benign tumour was an incidental finding.

Fig. 5.19 Gall stones in the common bile duct. M/73. This patient died from liver failure. The presence of the gall stones was not diagnosed during life.

Fig. 5.20 Calculus left in the common bile duct after cholecystectomy. M/73. During the operation the common bile duct was explored as can be seen by the ulceration in its lower part just proximal to the ampulla of Vater. A small gall stone, missed at the operation is impacted above the opening of the cystic duct near the bifurcation of the main hepatic ducts. The patient died a few days post-operatively from an acute myocardial infarction.

Fig. 5.21 Carcinoma of the gall bladder. F/74. A large calculus is present in the gall bladder. Tumour has extended into the adjacent liver.

Fig. 5.22 Adenocarcinoma arising from the bile ducts in the porta hepatis. F/78. The patient died from the effects of obstructive jaundice.

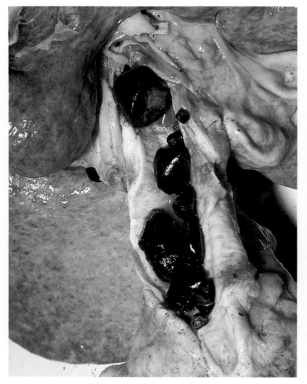

Fig. 5.19

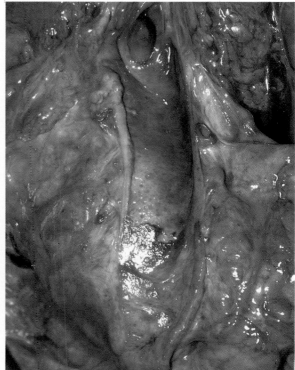

Fig. 5.20

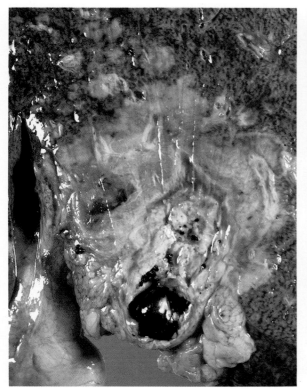

Fig. 5.21

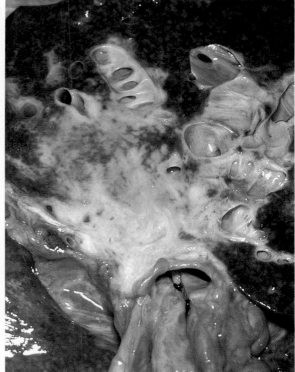

Fig. 5.22

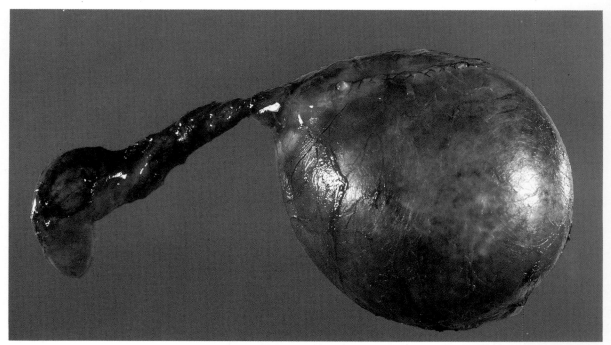

Fig. 5.23

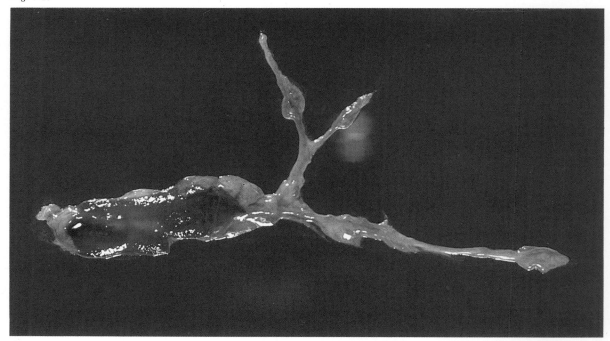

Fig. 5.24

Fig. 5.23 Choledochal cyst. F/5. The patient had been jaundiced since birth. At laparotomy this large cyst was found in the middle of the common bile duct and excised. The structure to the left is the attached gall bladder.

Fig. 5.24 Congenital biliary atresia. M/6. This child died from hepatic failure and the thin, stenosed extrahepatic biliary system was dissected. The right and left hepatic ducts and the common bile duct with the gall bladder attached on the left, are displayed. Sections showed the presence of only a microscopic lumen.

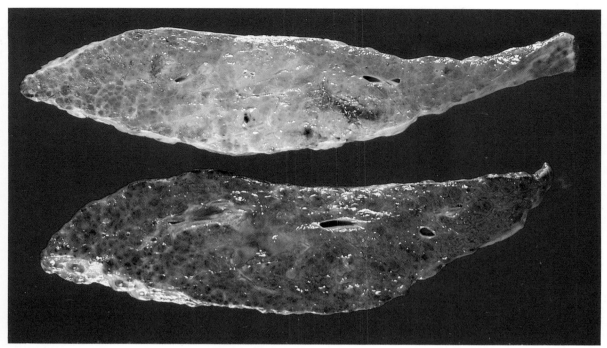

Fig. 5.25

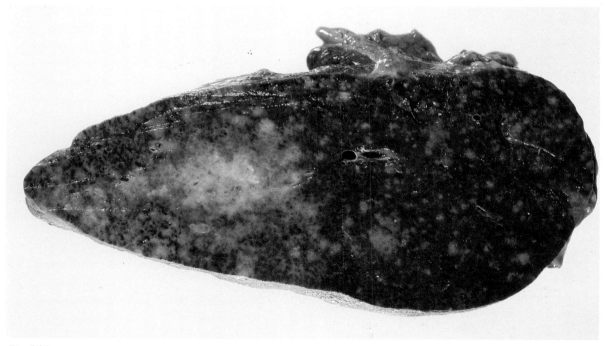

Fig. 5.26

Fig. 5.25 Haemochromatosis. M/70. This patient died from liver failure. The lower slice of liver shows cirrhosis. The deep brown colour is due to the deposition of iron, demonstrated in the upper slice which was stained with Prussian Blue solution.

Fig. 5.26 Haemochromatosis with hepatoma. M/59. There is a large hepatoma in the left lobe and multiple smaller foci of tumour throughout the liver.

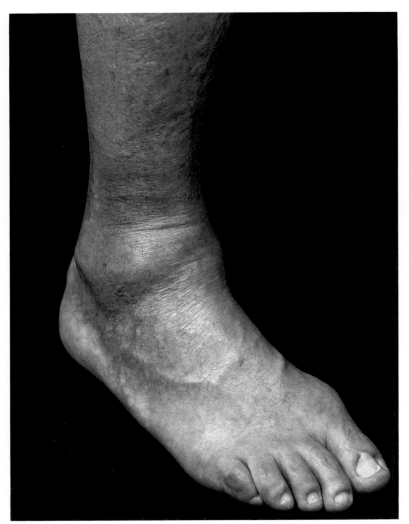

Fig. 5.27

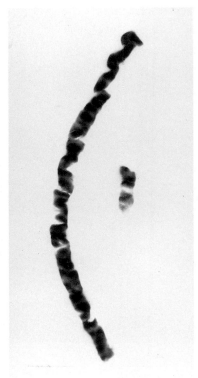

Fig. 5.29

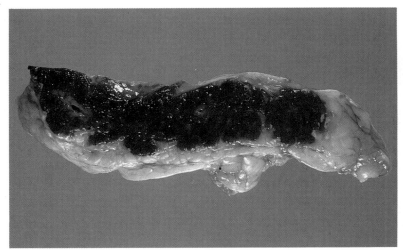

Fig. 5.28

Fig. 5.27 Arthritis in haemochromatosis. M/61. The brown pigmentation of the skin which is a feature of haemochromatosis can be seen, and the ankle joint is swollen. The arthritis is associated with the deposition of iron in the synovium of the joint.

Fig. 5.28 Pancreas in haemochromatosis. M/50. The pancreas is a red colour due to the deposition of iron. Diabetes is a common complication of haemochromatosis.

Fig. 5.29 Dubin Johnson Syndrome. M/20. This needle biopsy shows the black colour of the liver in this type of congenital hyperbilirubinaemia.

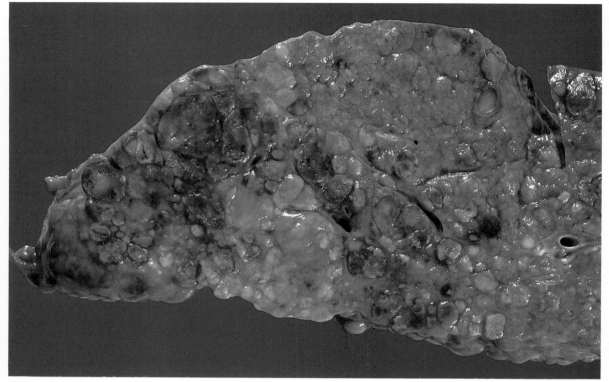

Fig. 5.30

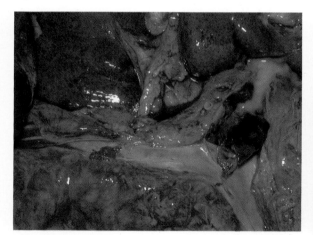

Fig. 5.31

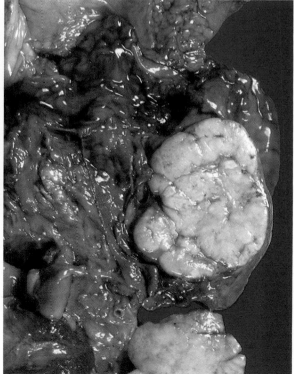

Fig. 5.32

Fig. 5.30 Hepatoma in macronodular cirrhosis. M/60. Both of these conditions are very common in the inhabitants of tropical countries. It is now thought that they are both caused by the hepatitis B virus. The multiple, brown nodules are tumour.

Fig. 5.31 Thrombosis of the portal vein. F/24. This is one of the complications of hepatoma.

Fig. 5.32 Secondary deposits of hepatoma in the lymph node in the porta hepatis. The common bile duct can be recognised to the left of the enlarged, tumour filled lymph node.

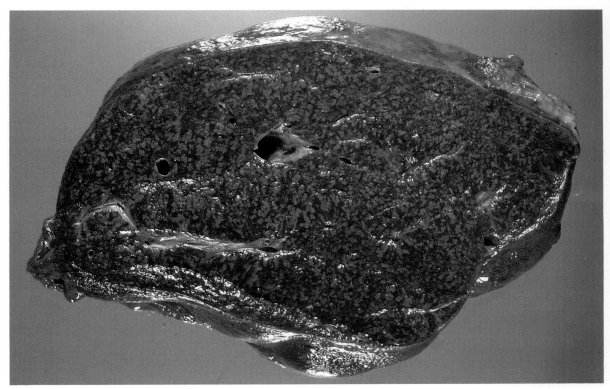

Fig. 5.33

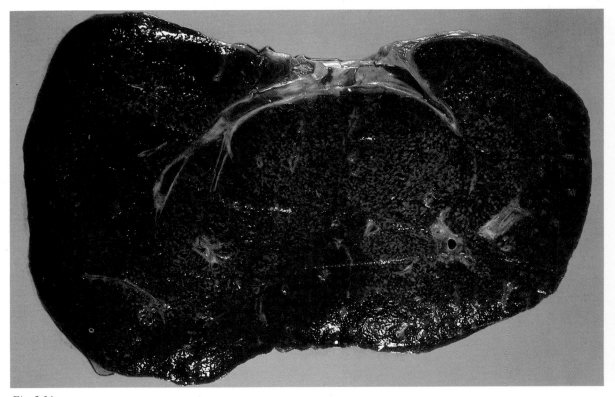

Fig. 5.34

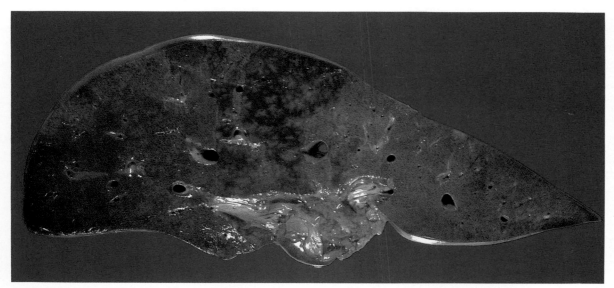

Fig. 5.35

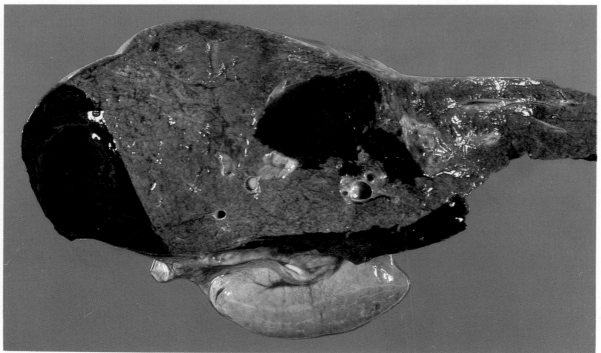

Fig. 5.36

Fig. 5.33 Liver showing the effects of long-standing cardiac failure resulting from a cardiomyopathy. M/35. The fibrosis in the region of the central hepatic veins can be recognised as multiple pale, irregular spots throughout the liver.

Fig. 5.34 Budd Chiari Syndrome. F/21. The liver has been sliced coronally with the caudate lobe in the middle. There is thrombus in the hepatic veins which resulted in venous congestion of the liver, most marked in the caudate lobe.

Fig. 5.35 Recent infarction in the liver. M/48. At post mortem there was a thrombus in the right hepatic artery.

Fig. 5.36 Subcapsular and intra hepatic haematoma. F/79. Bleeding had occurred from an intra hepatic vascular malformation. Such haematomas occur more frequently as a result of blunt trauma to the abdomen.

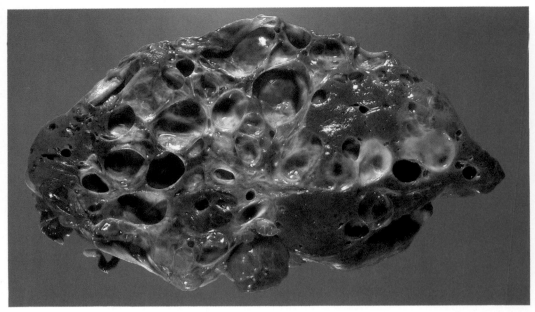

Fig. 5.37

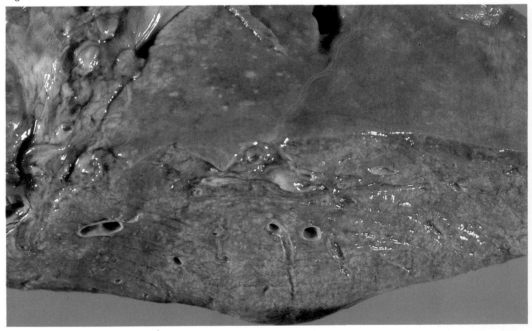

Fig. 5.38

Fig. 5.37 Congenital polycystic liver. M/54. This was associated with polycystic kidneys and the patient died from renal failure.

Fig. 5.38 Massive necrosis of the liver. F/67. The patient died three months after an attack of acute hepatitis. In the upper half of the specimen the capsule is intact and multiple, yellow areas can be seen through it. The lower half shows a cut surface. On the left there is an area of collapsed, atrophic liver and on the right, the yellow areas can be seen to be nodules of

regenerating liver cells. It was this appearance that gave rise to the name 'subacute yellow atrophy' for this condition.

Fig. 5.39 Suppurative cholangitis. F/45. The patient died from liver failure from extra hepatic obstruction caused by carcinoma of the head of the pancreas. The dilated bile ducts are filled with green, bile stained pus.

Fig. 5.40 Liver abscesses. F/87. This patient died from Gram-negative septicaemia and the abscesses are a complication of this. The site of the original infection was not found.

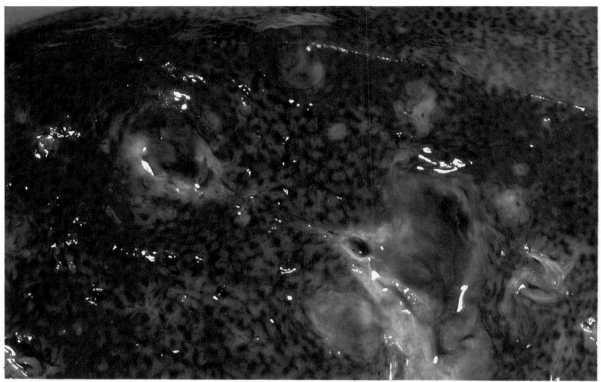

Fig. 5.39

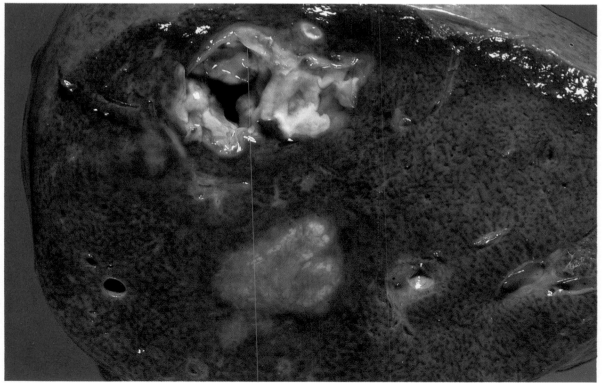

Fig. 5.40

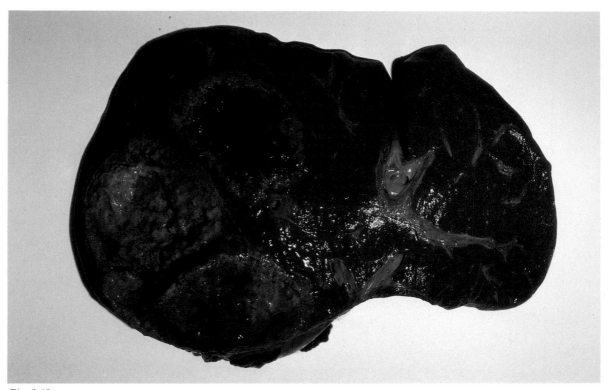

Fig. 5.45

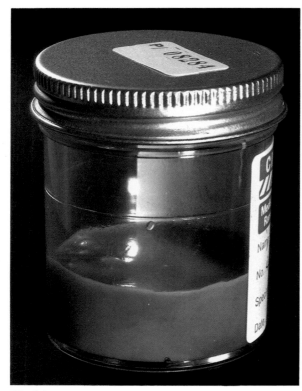

Fig. 5.46

Fig. 5.45 Amoebic abscess of the liver. M/49. There are three distinct loculi in this abscess which occupied most of the right lobe of the liver. The abscess was drained and a large amount of brown pus (anchovy sauce pus) was removed (Fig. 5.46). While undergoing treatment he suddenly developed pericardial effusion and died.

Fig. 5.46 Brown pus removed from the amoebic abscess of the liver shown in Fig. 5.45.

Fig. 5.47 Hydatid cyst of the liver. M/53. The patient had lived in a sheep raising area of Australia, but this was an incidental post mortem finding. The outer, thick fibrotic wall of the cyst is clearly seen and the cyst is filled with multiple daughter cysts of varying size.

Fig. 5.48 Clonorchis sinensis infestation of the liver. Korean seaman aged 35. The whole of the intra hepatic biliary system was filled with flukes. There is some thickening of the walls of the intra hepatic bile ducts but the infestation appeared to be essentially asymptomatic.

Fig. 5.49 Hepar lobatum. M/70. There was no other evidence of syphilis.

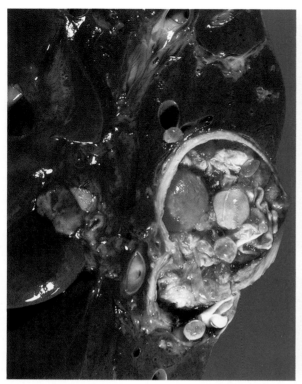

Fig. 5.47

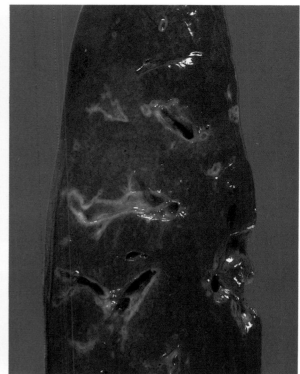

Fig. 5.48

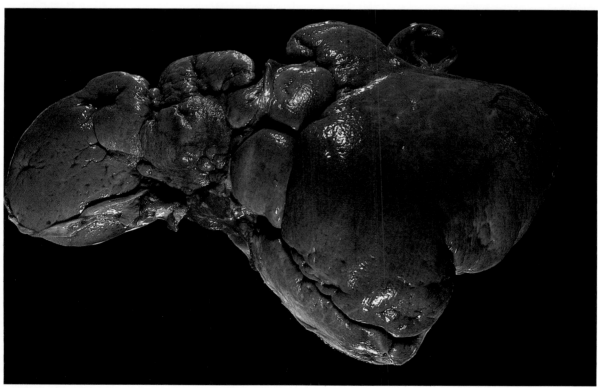

Fig. 5.49

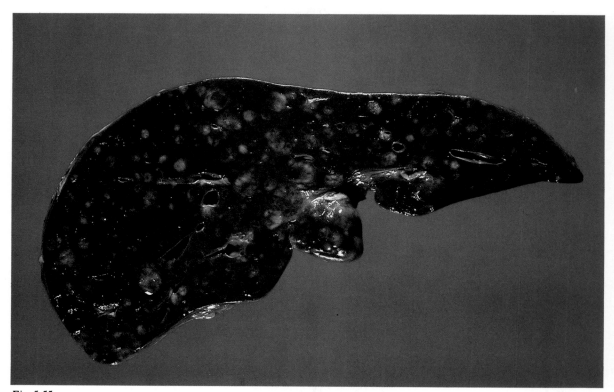

Fig. 5.55

Fig. 5.55 Secondary tumour in the liver. M/68. There are
multiple secondaries in both right and left lobes, and in the
caudate lobe. The primary was a bronchogenic carcinoma of
the lung.

6

Renal system

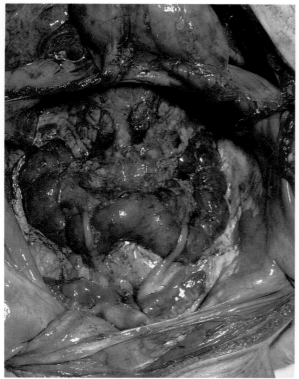

Fig. 6.1

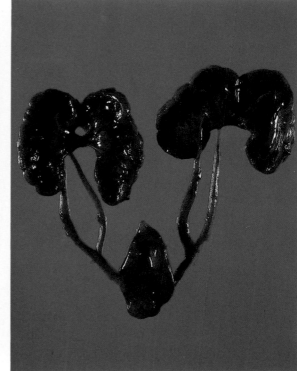

Fig. 6.2

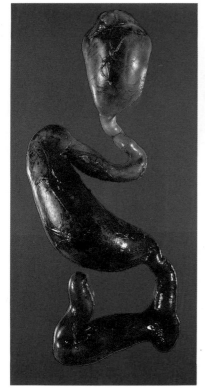

Fig. 6.3

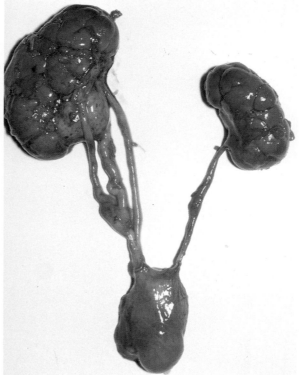

Fig. 6.4

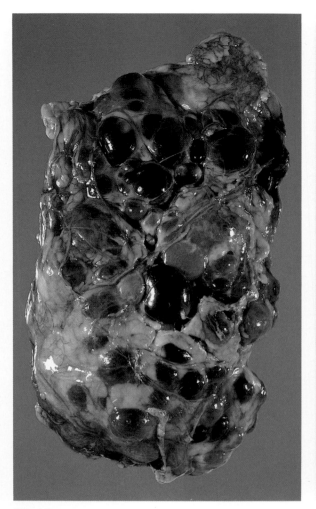

Fig. 6.5

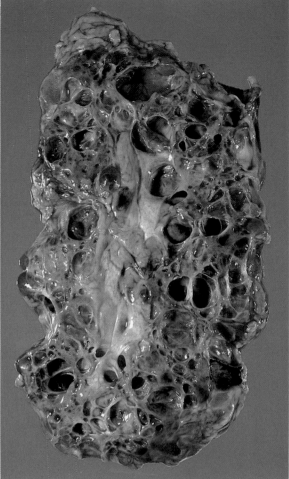

Fig. 6.6

Fig. 6.1 Horseshoe kidney. F/9 days. The lower poles of both kidneys are joined across the midline and the ureters pass anterior to the renal substance. This child died as a result of multiple congenital abnormalities.

Fig. 6.2 Double ureters. Neonate. Both ureters are bifid and join to form a single ureter before opening into the bladder.

Fig. 6.3 Megalouretar. M/11. This was caused by stenosis at the uretero-vesicle junction. The patient had recurrent urinary tract infections and finally the kidney and ureter were surgically removed.

Fig. 6.4 Triple ureter. Neonate. Double ureters are fairly common, but triple ureter is very rare.

Fig. 6.5 Polycystic disease of the kidneys. M/54. The kidney substance is almost completely replaced by cysts of varying size. The kidneys may be not much bigger than normal, but usually they are quite large.

Fig. 6.6 Cut surface of specimen in Fig. 6.5 showing the cysts with very little normal renal tissue remaining. Polycystic kidneys characteristically cause symptoms after the age of 40.

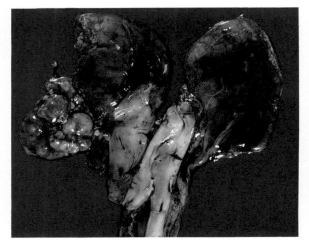

Fig. 6.7

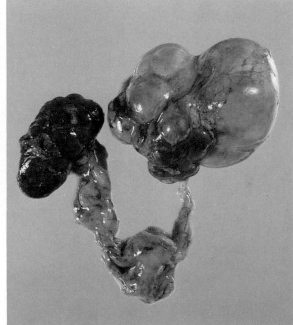

Fig. 6.8

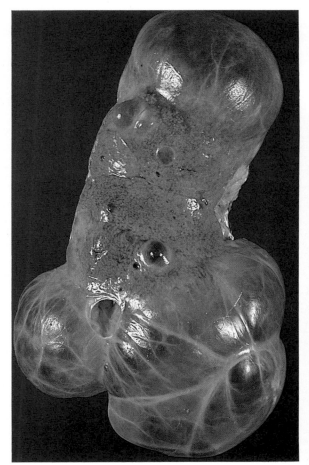

Fig. 6.9

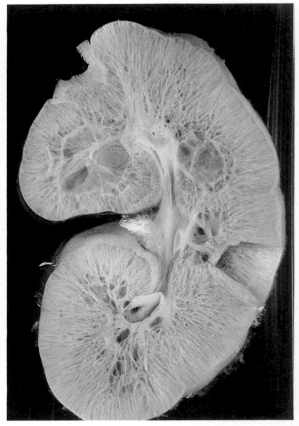

Fig. 6.10

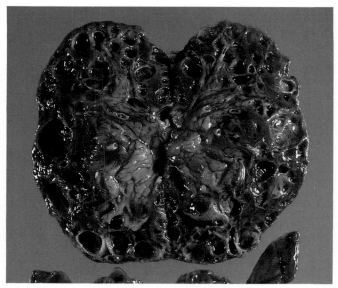

Fig. 6.11

Fig. 6.7 Cystic dysplastic kidney. Stillborn. There is a very small multicystic kidney on the right and no kidney on the left. The adrenal glands are relatively large in neonates, but they are accentuated in this case because of the very small size of the kidney.

Fig. 6.8 Cystic dysplastic kidney. F/24 hours. The right kidney is normal but the left is grossly cystic. Microscopic examination showed malformed renal substance together with areas of cartilage. Cystic dysplastic kidney may be unilateral or bilateral.

Fig. 6.9 Multiple simple cysts in the kidney. M/70. This was an incidental post mortem finding.

Fig. 6.10 Sponge kidney in a neonate who died a few minutes after birth. This type of cystic kidney is usually large and bilateral and may interfere with delivery of the foetus.

Fig. 6.11 Multicystic kidneys resulting from long-term haemodialysis for chronic renal disease. M/68.

Fig. 6.12 Hydatid cyst of the kidney. M/10. The unruptured, white laminated membrane of the cyst can be seen in the upper pole. It had compressed the calyceal system causing hydronephrosis. The kidney was removed because the clinical and radiological features resembled those of a primary renal tumour. There was no history of exposure to sheep farming.

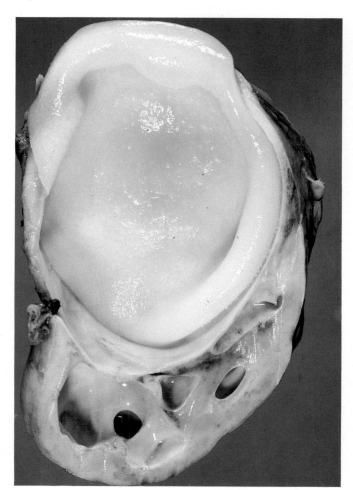

Fig. 6.12

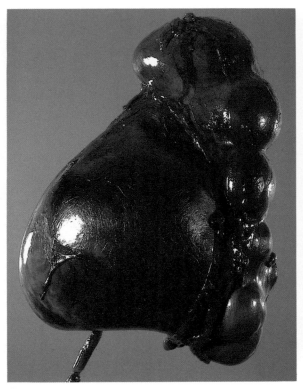

Fig. 6.13

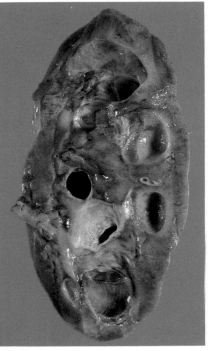

Fig. 6.14

Fig. 6.13 Hydronephrosis due to congenital pelviureteric obstruction. F/46. There is marked dilatation of the renal pelvis and atrophy of renal substance. The upper end of the ureter is atrophic and its lumen was microscopic. The patient had experienced no symptoms until just prior to the nephrectomy when she presented with abdominal pain.

Fig. 6.14 Hydronephrosis. F/73. There is marked dilatation of all of the calyces with atrophy of the renal papillae. These are the results of ureteric obstruction which in this case was caused by a transitional cell carcinoma of the bladder.

Fig. 6.15 'Uric acid infarcts'. Neonate. The yellow streaks in the renal papillae are due to deposition of uric acid crystals. This does not appear to have any clinical significance.

Fig. 6.16 Multiple renal cortical infarcts. M/15 months. The creamy areas of infarction are surrounded by areas of haemorrhage. The renal damage resulted from a sudden drop in blood pressure following haemorrhage.

Fig. 6.17 Renal tubular necrosis. M/8 weeks. The tubular necrosis is shown by the presence of haemorrhagic streaking in the medulla and renal papillae. It was a complication of peritonitis.

Fig. 6.18 Infarction of the kidney due to thrombosis of the renal vein. M/10 months. The whole kidney was infarcted. The child was severely dehydrated from gastroenteritis. Thrombosis of renal, pulmonary or cerebral veins may occur as a complication of dehydration in children.

Fig. 6.19 Infarction of the kidney caused by thrombosis of a large branch of the renal artery. M/55. The infarcted area has become discoloured and depressed below the adjacent kidney surface. The thrombus was a complication of atherosclerosis of the renal artery.

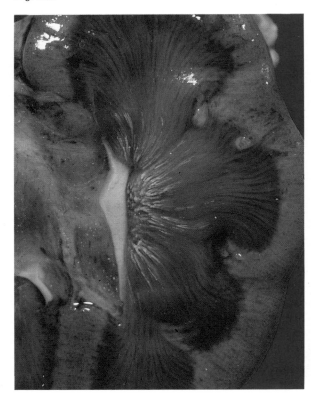

Fig. 6.15

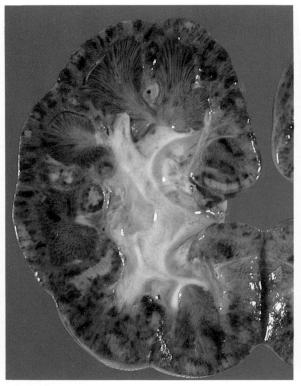

Fig. 6.16

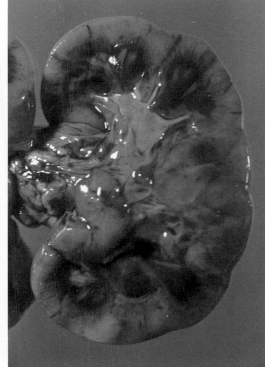

Fig. 6.17

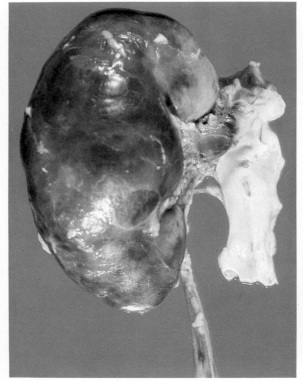

Fig. 6.18

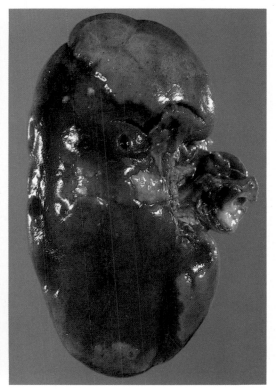

Fig. 6.19

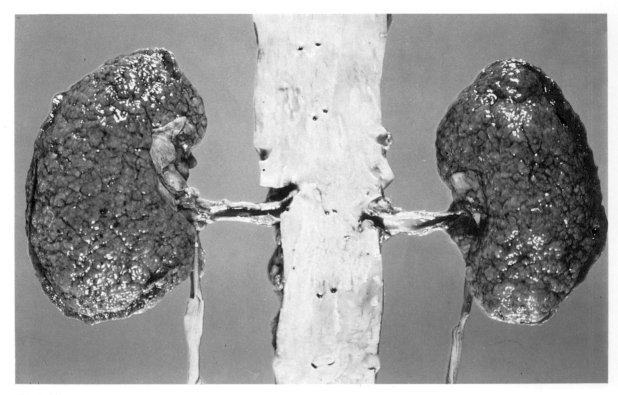

Fig. 6.20

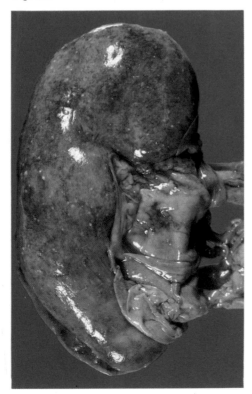

Fig. 6.21

Fig. 6.20 Benign nephrosclerosis. M/70. Both kidneys are slightly reduced in size, the result of atherosclerosis of the renal arteries.

Fig. 6.21 Acute pyelonephritis. F/71. The outer surface of the kidney shows multiple, creamy spots. These are abscesses and when the capsule is stripped from the cortical surface, pus is released from the most superficial of them.

Fig. 6.22 Acute pyelonephritis. M/58. The cut surface of the kidney shows reddening of the mucosa of the calyceal system. There are multiple yellow abscesses throughout the renal cortex which itself appears to be hyperaemic.

Fig. 6.23 Diabetic kidneys with pyelonephritis and papillary necrosis. M/47. Infection is an important complication of diabetes and renal infection may sometimes cause death as in this case.

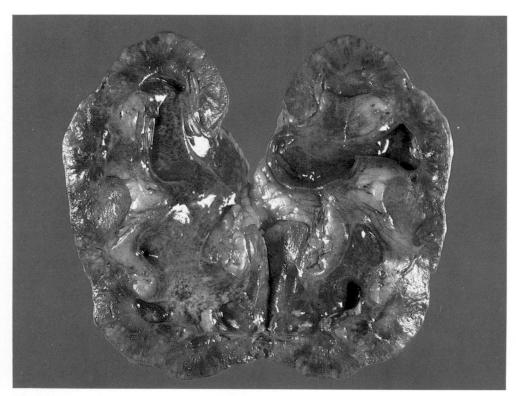

Fig. 6.22

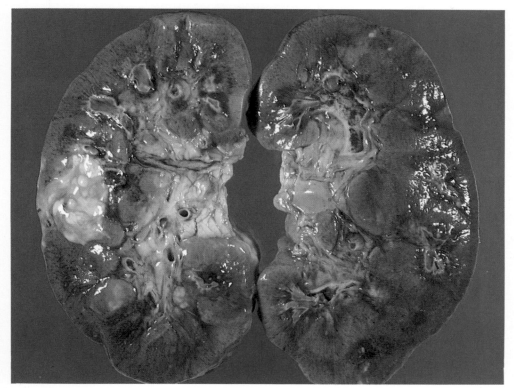

Fig. 6.23

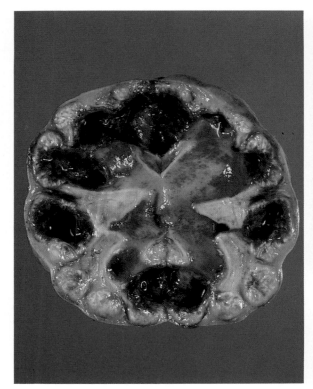

Fig. 6.24

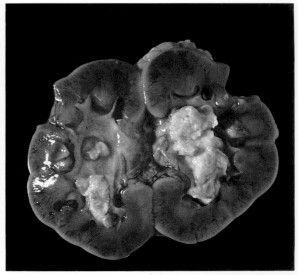

Fig. 6.25

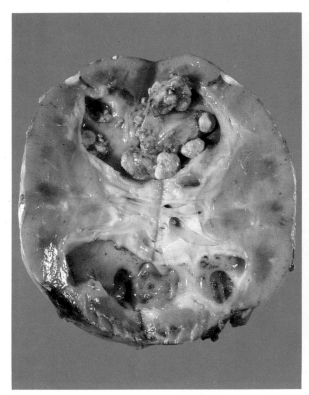

Fig. 6.26

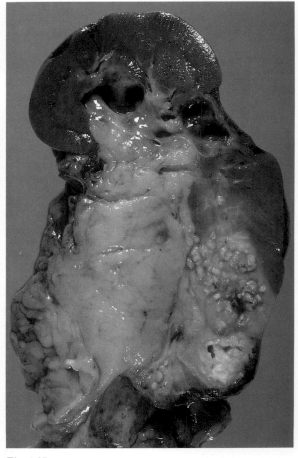

Fig. 6.27

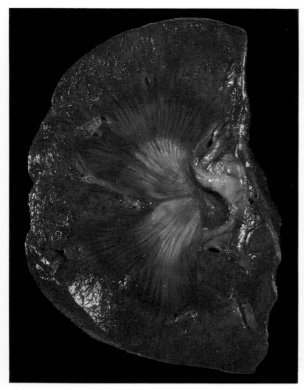

Fig. 6.28

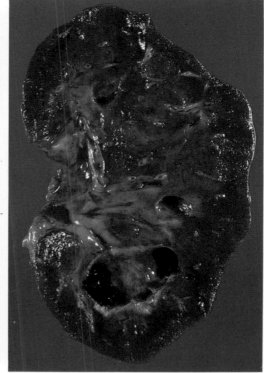

Fig. 6.29

Fig. 6.24 Xanthogranulomatous pyelonephritis. F/60. The kidney is opened to show the features of acute pyelonephritis already displayed in Fig. 6.22 together with large areas of haemorrhage and lipid accumulation. These features occur in a small percentage of cases of pyelonephritis, but do not appear to have any special significance.

Fig. 6.25 Pyonephrosis. M/26 weeks. This child had congenital abnormalities of the lower urinary tract which predisposed to infection. As well as acute pyelonephritis there is a large amount of pus in the calyceal system.

Fig. 6.26 Nephrolithiasis and hydronephrosis. F/42. Fragments of a staghorn calculus are impacted in the calyces at the upper pole of the kidney.

Fig. 6.27 Renal tuberculosis. M/28. In the lower third of the kidney there is a caseous inflammatory mass extending through the whole thickness of the renal cortex. Numerous acid fast bacilli were demonstrated in the microscopic sections.

Fig. 6.28 Early analgesic nephropathy. F/54. There is a heavy deposition of lipid in the renal papilla. The remainder of the kidney is still relatively normal.

Fig. 6.29 More advanced analgesic nephropathy. M/60. There is acute necrosis of the renal papillae especially in the lower pole, and shrinkage and scarring of the renal substance is beginning.

Fig. 6.30 Advanced analgesic nephropathy. F/41. The kidneys are small and irregularly scarred. The renal papillae have virtually all disappeared and the cortex is very thin.

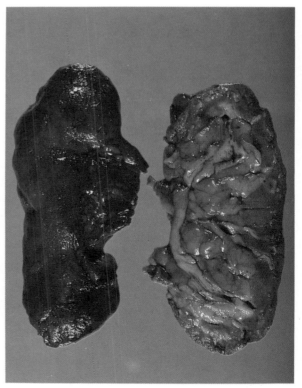

Fig. 6.30

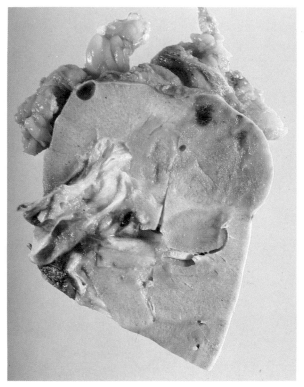

Fig. 6.31

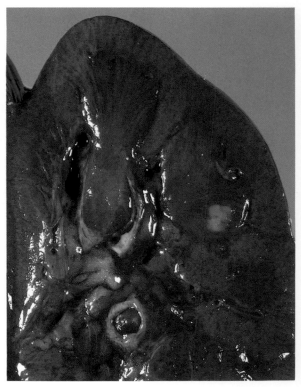

Fig. 6.32

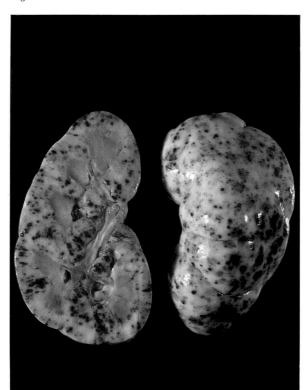

Fig. 6.33

Fig. 6.31 Oncocytoma (renal tubular adenoma) F/79. There is a well circumscribed, homogeneous, brown tumour in the renal cortex. These tumours are benign but this kidney was removed because of a radiological diagnosis of renal carcinoma.

Fig. 6.32 Intramedullary fibroma. F/58. This is a small, pale, benign tumour which causes no clinical symptoms and is frequently found in examination of post mortem kidneys.

Fig. 6.33 Kidneys in acute lymphoblastic leukaemia. F/3. The kidneys are pale because of the anaemia. The normal architecture has been replaced by an infiltration of creamy, haemorrhagic tissue. The kidneys have been enlarged by this infiltrate.

Fig. 6.34 Wilm's tumour. F/5. The tumour occupies the whole upper pole of the kidney. Its cut surface shows some firm, homogeneous areas and other areas of necrosis.

Fig. 6.35 Adenocarcinoma of the kidney (Grawitz tumour). F/36. Most of the kidney has been replaced by tumour which has extended through the capsule. The tumour has a variegated appearance with some solid and some cystic areas. The renal vein in the hilum is filled with tumour.

Fig. 6.36 Transitional cell carcinoma of the renal pelvis. These tumours frequently have a papilliferous appearance.

Fig. 6.37 Transitional cell carcinoma of the ureter. M/52. This tumour is more solid and less papillary than the one illustrated in Fig. 6.36. It caused obstruction and the ureter proximal to the tumour has become somewhat dilated.

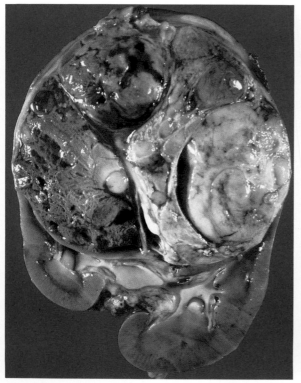

Fig. 6.34

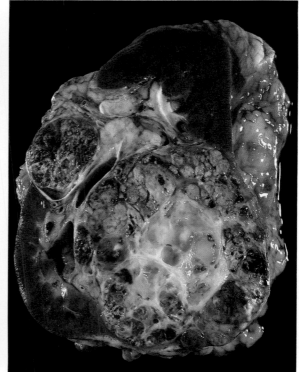

Fig. 6.35

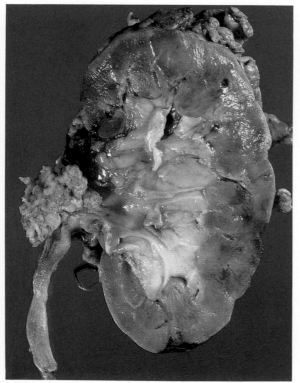

Fig. 6.36

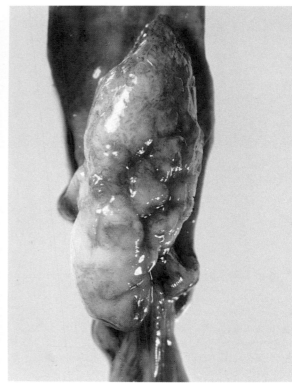

Fig. 6.37

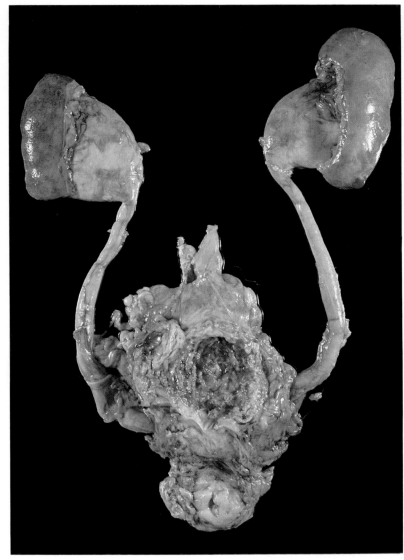

Fig. 6.38

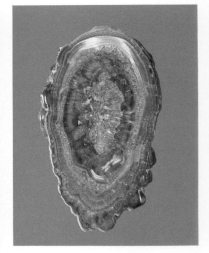

Fig. 6.39

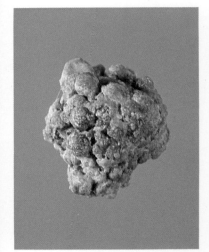

Fig. 6.40

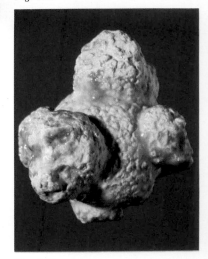

Fig. 6.41

Fig. 6.38 Carcinoma of the bladder. M/88. The entire mucosal surface is replaced by a transitional cell carcinoma. It has caused obstruction with bilateral hydro-ureter and hydronephrosis.

Fig. 6.39 Renal calculus which has been cut and its surface polished to show its laminations.

Fig. 6.40 Ureteric calculus.

Fig. 6.41 Bossellated vesical calculus.

7

Male genital system

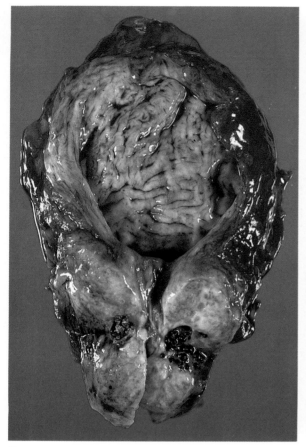

Fig. 7.1

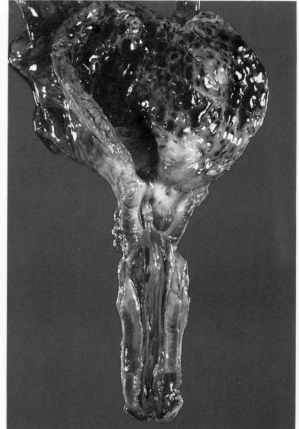

Fig. 7.2

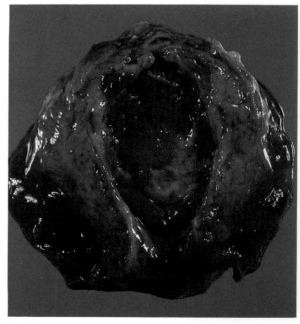

Fig. 7.3

Fig. 7.1 Benign prostatic hypertrophy. M/84. The prostate is considerably enlarged. Its cut surface shows a creamy, lobulated appearance. There are a number of calculi in the prostatic ducts. The middle lobe has extended into the base of the bladder and the longstanding prostatic obstruction has caused thickening and trabeculation of the bladder wall.

Fig. 7.2 Bladder outlet obstruction caused by posterior urethral valves. M/6. This boy had suffered from repeated attacks of urinary tract infection since birth and died during one of these episodes. The valves can be seen arising from the verumontanum. The bladder is hypertrophied and the mucosal surface is grossly trabeculated.

Fig. 7.3 Acute cystitis. F/36. The mucosal surface is red and inflamed. The patient had an indwelling catheter for many weeks before death from other pathology.

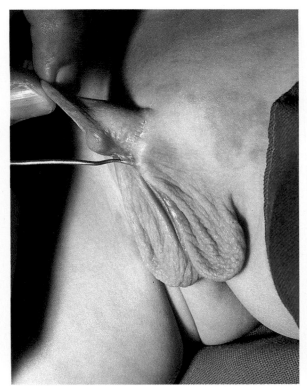

Fig. 7.4

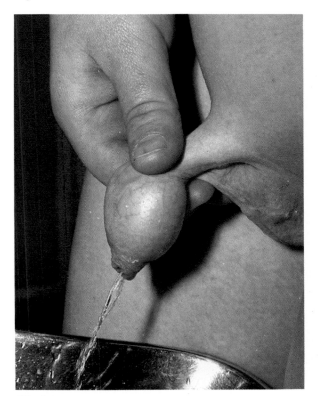

Fig. 7.5

Fig. 7.4 Hypospadias. M/1. The urethra opens at the base of the penis. The penis itself is short and bent.

Fig. 7.5 Epispadias. M/2.

Fig. 7.6 Phimosis. M/8. This is caused by partial stenosis of the prepuce. Urine collects under the prepuce during micturition.

Fig. 7.6

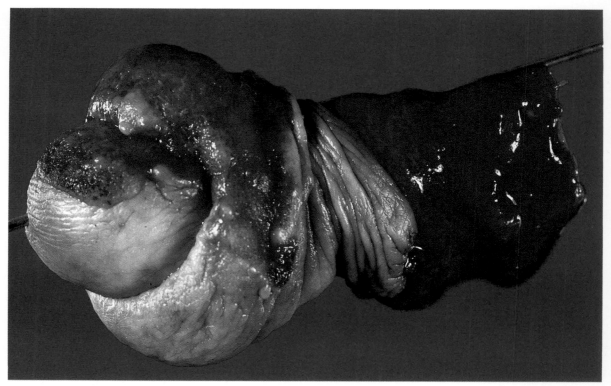

Fig. 7.7

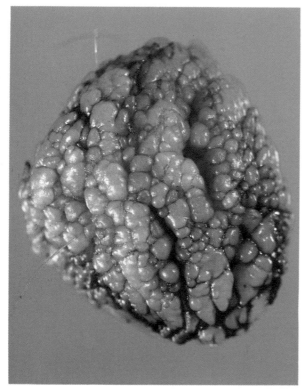

Fig. 7.7 Squamous cell carcinoma of the penis. M/69. There is an ulcerating squamous cell carcinoma eroding the prepuce and the dorsal surface of the glans.

Fig. 7.8 Condylomata accuminata of perineum. M/55. These are thought to be viral induced and can occur in the ano-genital region of both males and females. They are treated by simple excision.

Fig. 7.9 Torsion of the testis. M/14 days. The testis is swollen, black and necrotic. The twist in the cord is demonstrated. When this occurs in babies, it presents as a lump in the scrotum. In adults it presents with sudden onset of severe pain.

Fig. 7.10 Hydrocoele. M/3 months. The tunica vaginalis is filled with clear fluid. In children, the tunica still retains its connection with the abdominal cavity.

Fig. 7.11 Chronic hydrocoele. M/56. In adults, the tunica vaginalis has lost its connection with the abdominal cavity and fluid collects locally. As time passes, the tunica becomes fibrotic and sometimes calcifies.

Fig. 7.8

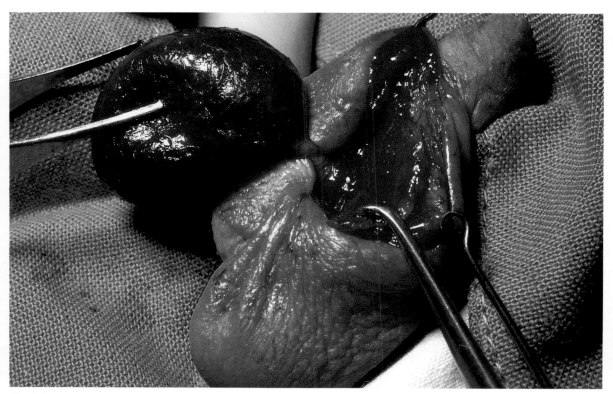

Fig. 7.9

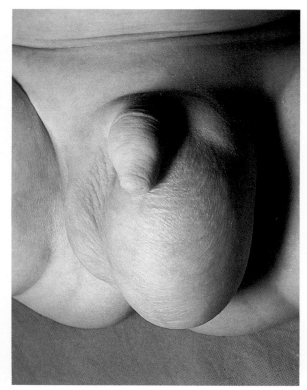

Fig. 7.10

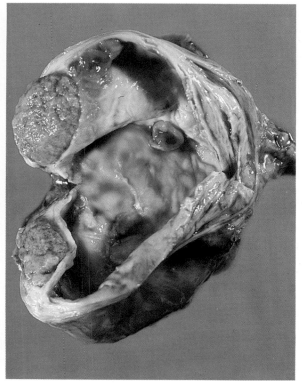

Fig. 7.11

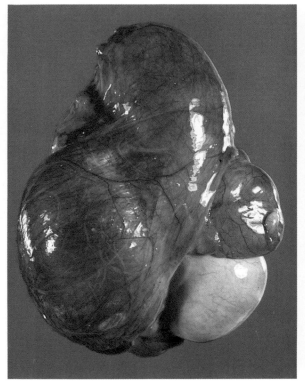

Fig. 7.12

Fig. 7.13

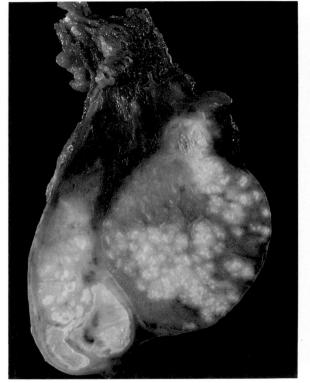

Fig. 7.14

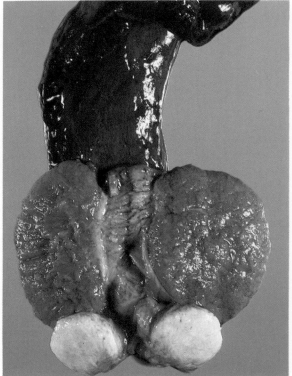

Fig. 7.15

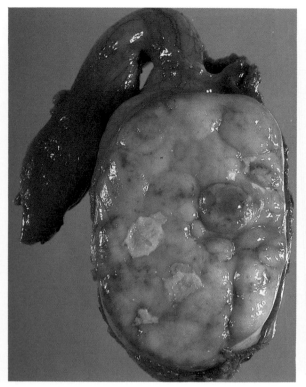

Fig. 7.16

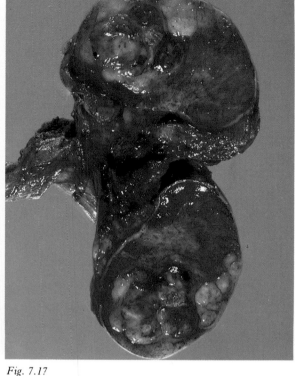

Fig. 7.17

Fig. 7.12 Cyst of the epididymis. M/34. The cyst is multiloculated and filled with clear fluid. It develops behind the testis.

Fig. 7.13 Abscess in the epididymis. M/78. Thick purulent material is replacing the epididymis. The patient presented with a mass in the scrotum.

Fig. 7.14 Tuberculosis of the testis and epididymis. M/23. The testis contains multiple, rounded granulomatous lesions. The epididymis is almost completely replaced by similar tissue. The patient had disseminated tuberculosis.

Fig. 7.15 Adenomatoid tumour of the epididymis. M/54. There is a creamy, well circumscribed tumour in the epididymis.

Fig. 7.16 Seminoma of the testis. M/40. The testis is enlarged and completely replaced by fleshy, lobulated, homogeneous, creamy tissue.

Fig. 7.17 Combined teratoma and seminoma of the testis. M/20. The cut surface of this tumour shows some areas which are homogeneous (the seminoma), and other areas that are necrotic and haemorrhagic (the teratoma).

Fig. 7.18 Regressing seminoma of the testis. M/26. This man died from disseminated malignancy. The main bulk of the tumour involved the para-aortic and mediastinal lymph nodes, and there were pulmonary secondaries. After careful slicing of both testes this small, creamy focus of tumour was found. Microscopically it consisted of small numbers of seminoma cells surrounded by an inflammatory cell reaction.

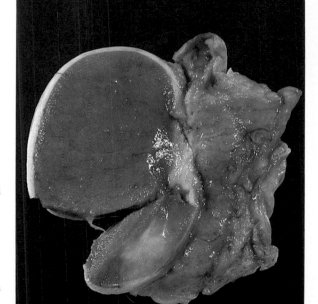

Fig. 7.18

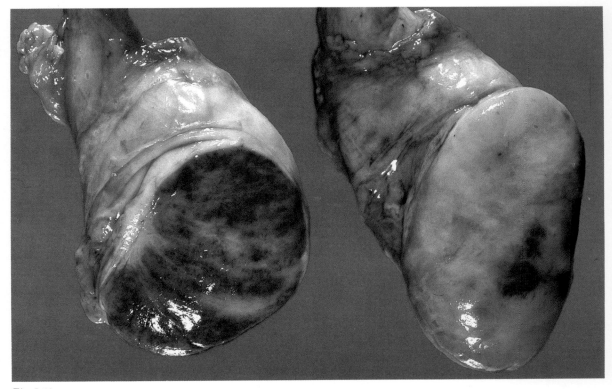

Fig. 7.19

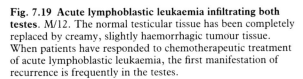

Fig. 7.19 Acute lymphoblastic leukaemia infiltrating both testes. M/12. The normal testicular tissue has been completely replaced by creamy, slightly haemorrhagic tumour tissue. When patients have responded to chemotherapeutic treatment of acute lymphoblastic leukaemia, the first manifestation of recurrence is frequently in the testes.

Fig. 7.20 Infantile embryonal carcinoma. M/9 months. The tumour has a homogeneous, creamy cut surface and has completely replaced the normal testicular tissue. This is the special type of malignant tumour of the testis that occurs in children. Its old name was orchioblastoma.

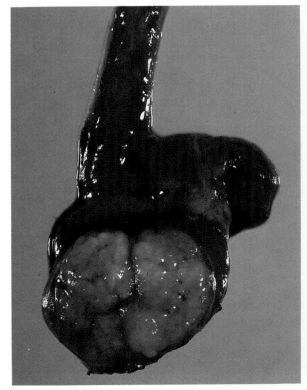

Fig. 7.20

8

Breast and female genital system

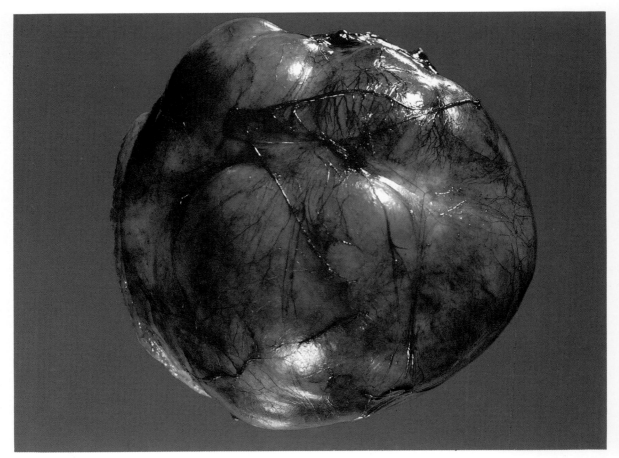

Fig. 8.1

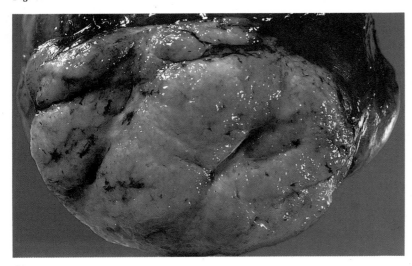

Fig. 8.2

Fig. 8.1 Fibroadenoma. F/18. This well circumscribed and mobile nodule was removed surgically.

Fig. 8.2 Cut surface of Fig. 8.1 showing a lobulated appearance. The tissue bulges outwards.

Fig. 8.3 Mammary duct ectasia. F/55. Lump removed from just below the nipple. When cut across it showed many dilated ducts filled with cheesy material, some of which can be seen on the right of the specimen.

Fig. 8.4 Intraduct papilloma. F/67. Presented with bleeding from the nipple associated with a breast lump. A large breast duct has been opened and it contains a fleshy tumour arising from its wall.

Fig. 8.5 Fibrocystic disease of the breast. F/35. The breast lump shows multiple small, blue coloured, fluid filled cysts. The adjacent breast tissue is somewhat fibrous.

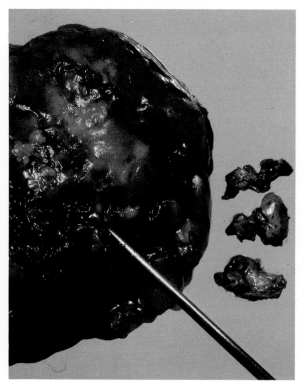

Fig. 8.3

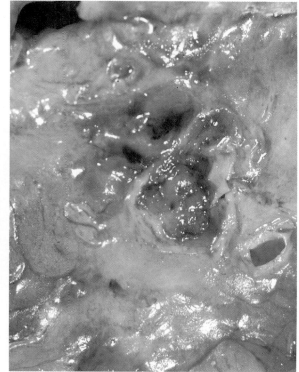

Fig. 8.4

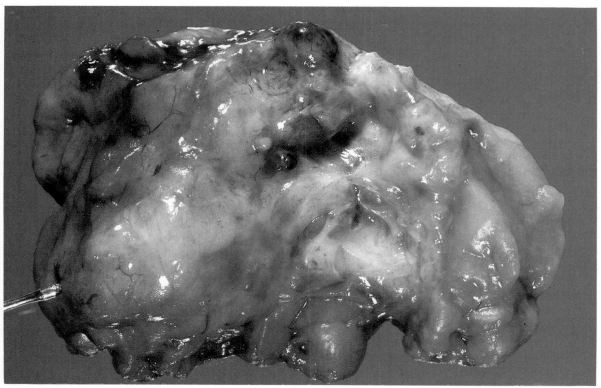

Fig. 8.5

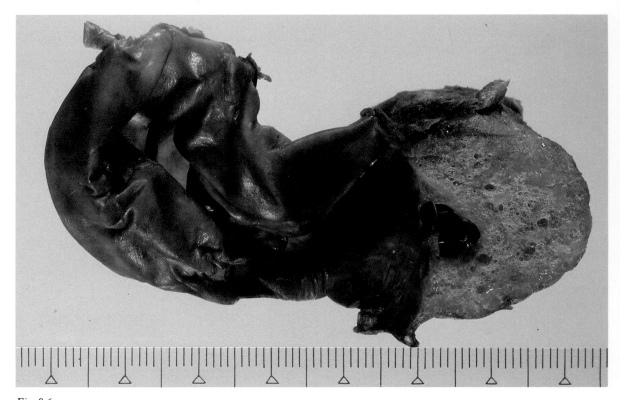

Fig. 8.6

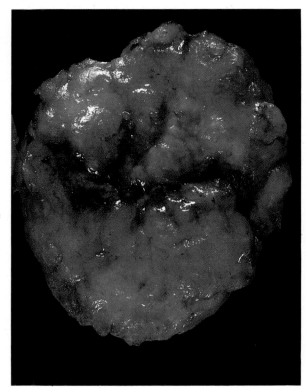

Fig. 8.6 Lipogranuloma caused by rupture of a polythene, paraffin-filled sac implanted some 30 years previously as a device for breast augmentation. F/47.

Fig. 8.7 Fat necrosis. F/42. Note the variegated colour and areas of haemorrhage on the cut surface of this lump. It was gritty to cut due to the presence of spotty calcification.

Fig. 8.8 Carcinoma of the left breast. F/60. A small lump was palpable and when the hands were raised above the head, tethering to the skin was accentuated.

Fig. 8.9 Carcinoma of the breast. F/70. A breast lump removed for frozen section. When cut across, it was hard and gritty and the cut surface bulged inwards.

Fig. 8.10 Carcinoma of the breast. F/35. A larger lump than in Fig. 8.9 but again showing inward bulging.

Fig. 8.7

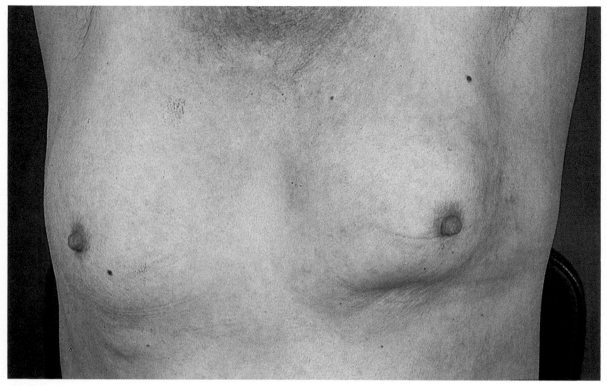

Fig. 8.8

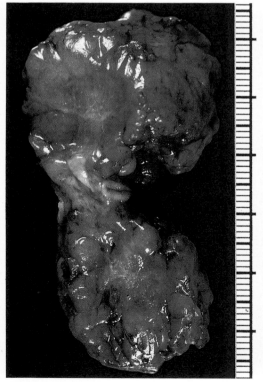

Fig. 8.9

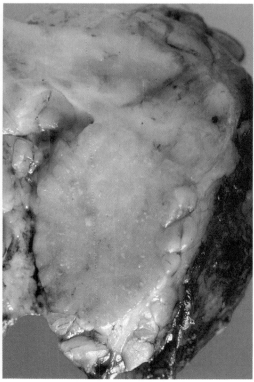

Fig. 8.10

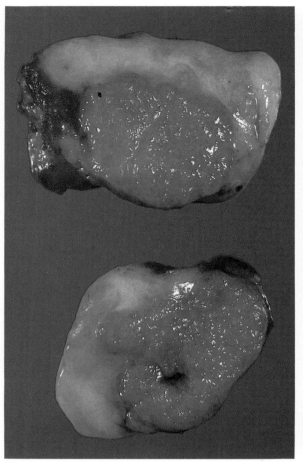

Fig. 8.11

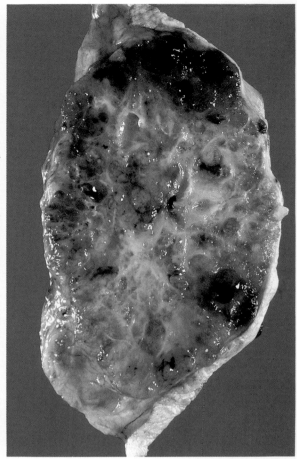

Fig. 8.12

Fig. 8.11 Medullary carcinoma of the breast. F/50. Well circumscribed, soft breast lump. The diagnosis of carcinoma was confirmed on microscopic examination.

Fig. 8.12 Colloid carcinoma of the breast. F/70. This is a large tumour and the cut surface has an extremely mucoid appearance.

Fig. 8.13 Paget's Disease of the nipple. F/66. The crusted, eroded surface is characteristic of this condition. There is always an associated carcinoma present in the breast.

Fig. 8.14 Extramammary Paget's Disease of the scrotum. M/58. Note the red, scaling skin. The commonest site for extramammary Paget's disease is the ano-genital region in both sexes. Only a small proportion of cases have carcinoma in the underlying apocrine glands.

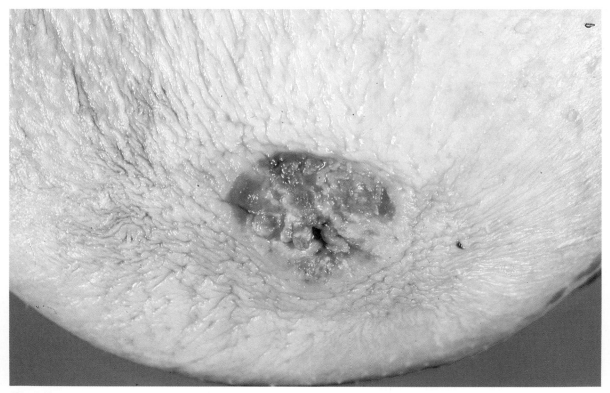

Fig. 8.13

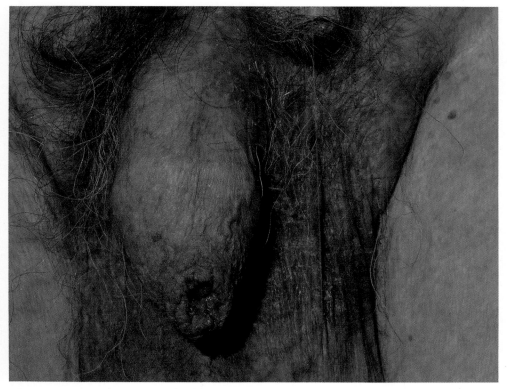

Fig. 8.14

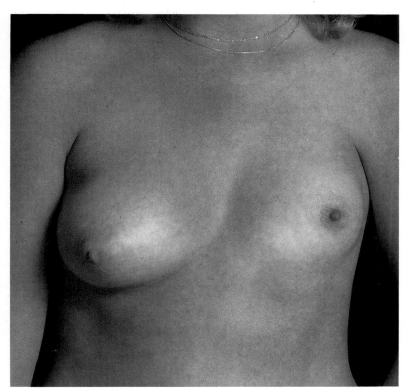

Fig. 8.15

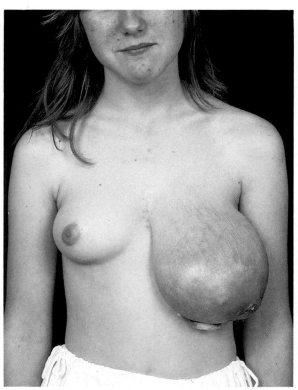

Fig. 8.16

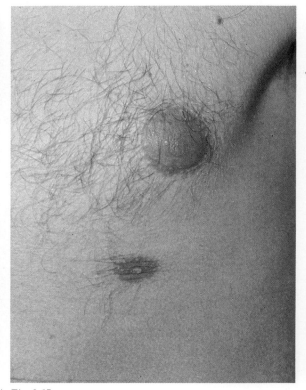

Fig. 8.17

Fig. 8.15 Congenital hypoplasia of the left breast. F/18.

Fig. 8.16 Juvenile hypertrophy of the left breast. F/13. The redness is due to local cellulitis from ulceration caused by wearing a bra that was too tight. The benign tumorous tissue was removed and the breast was reconstructed.

Fig. 8.17 Accessory nipple. M/23.

Fig. 8.18 Carcinoma of the right breast. M/55. There is already ulceration of the skin in spite of the fact that the tumour is quite small. Cancer of the male breast is rare and is often advanced at the time of first presentation.

Fig. 8.19 Gynaecomastia. M/20.

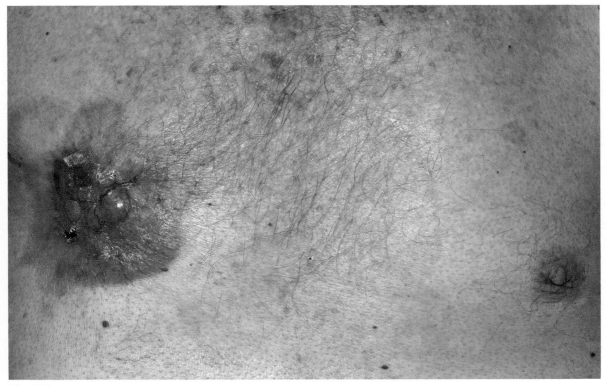

Fig. 8.18

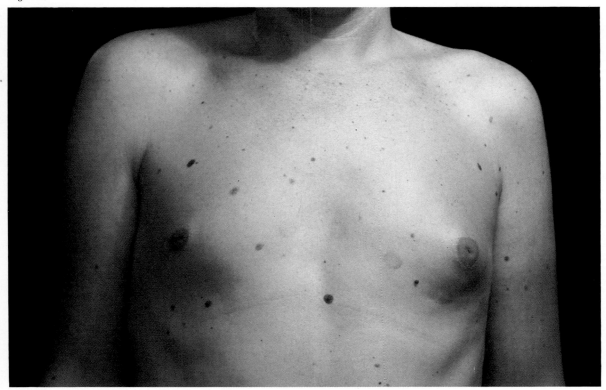

Fig. 8.19

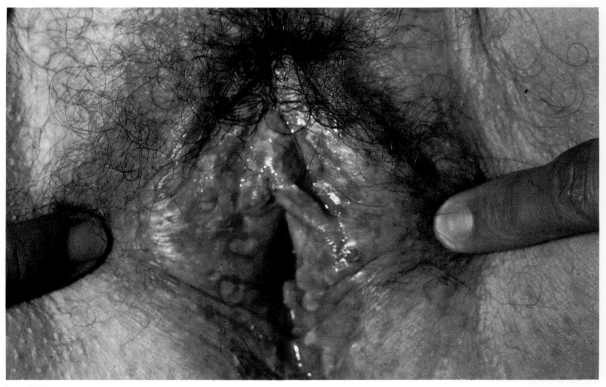

Fig. 8.20

Fig. 8.20 Acute vulvitis. F/40. The exact cause can only be determined by the results of bacteriological culture.

Fig. 8.21 Condylomata lata. F/20. Spirochaetes were seen in dark ground microscopic examination of smears from the lesions. Serological tests for syphilis were positive.

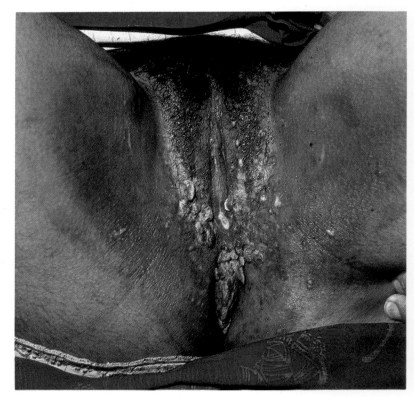

Fig. 8.21

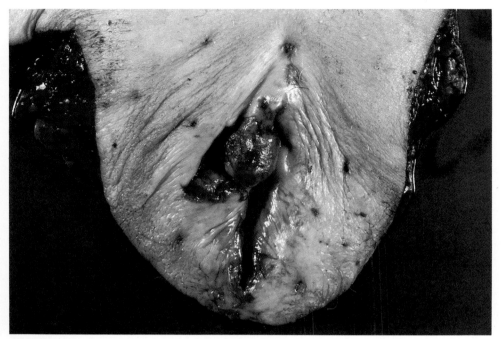

Fig. 8.22

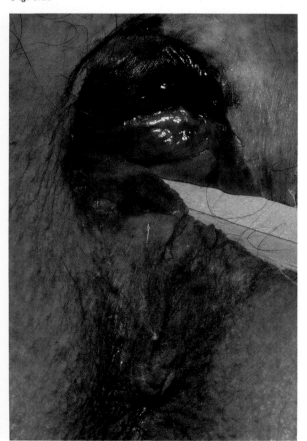

Fig. 8.22 Squamous cell carcinoma arising from the right labium minus. F/79. Treated by radical vulvectomy.

Fig. 8.23 Malignant melanoma in the vagina. F/78.

Fig. 8.23

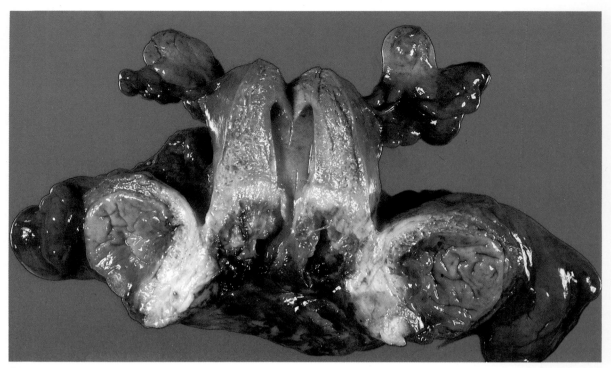

Fig. 8.24

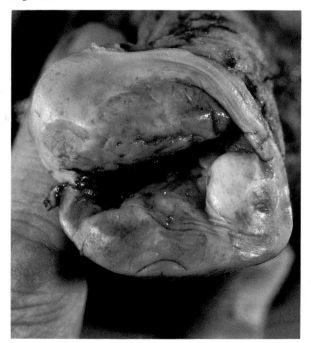

Fig. 8.25

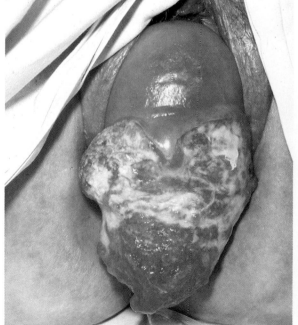

Fig. 8.26

Fig. 8.24 Advanced squamous cell carcinoma of the cervix. F/41. The panhysterectomy specimen shows that the cervix has been completely eroded by a malignant neoplasm.

Fig. 8.25 Carcinoma in situ plus early invasive squamous cell

carcinoma of the cervix. F/41. The cervix is eroded. The diagnosis was made on Papanicolau smear and biopsy.

Fig. 8.26 Squamous cell carcinoma arising in a longstanding procidentia. F/72.

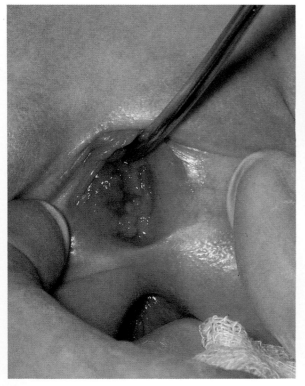

Fig. 8.27

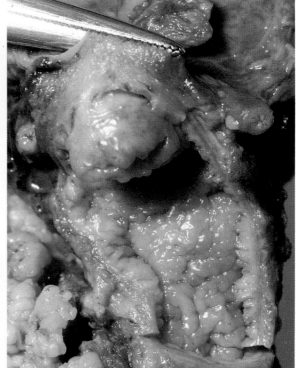

Fig. 8.28

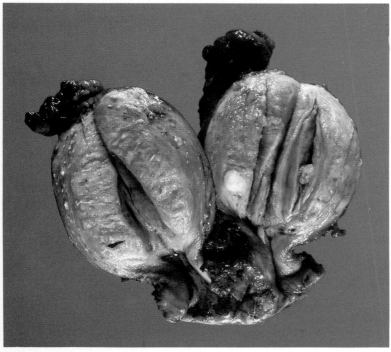

Fig. 8.29

Fig. 8.27 Embryonal rhabdomyosarcoma. F/2. The mother noticed soft nodules protruding from the vagina.

Fig. 8.28 Pelvic exenteration was performed on the patient in Fig. 8.27. Soft tumour masses can be seen covering the vagina and cervix—the so-called Botryoid Sarcoma.

Fig. 8.29 Double uterus.

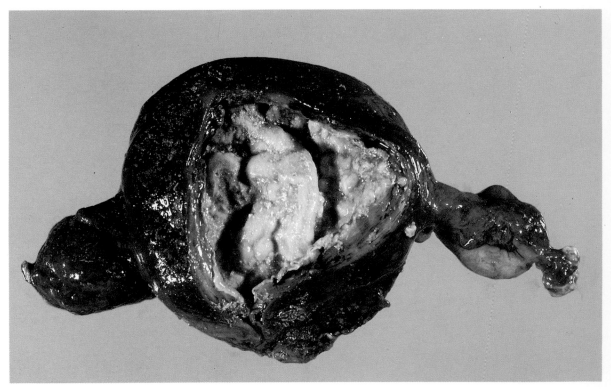

Fig. 8.30

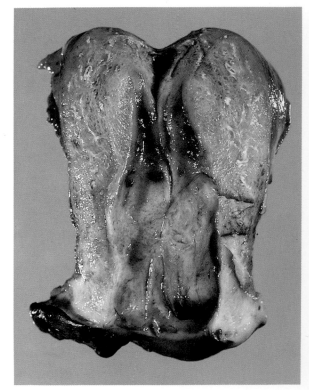

Fig. 8.30 Pyometra. F/67. There is cervical stenosis and the uterine cavity is filled with pus.

Fig. 8.31 Benign endometrial polyp. F/37. The soft polyp was attached to the endometrium. The patient presented with menorrhagia.

Fig. 8.31

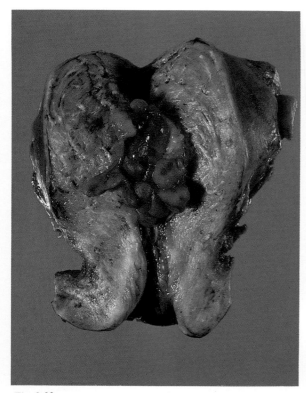

Fig. 8.32

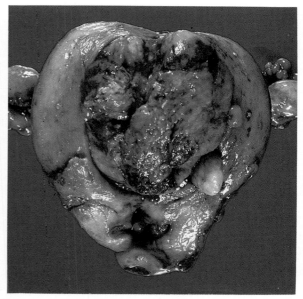

Fig. 8.33

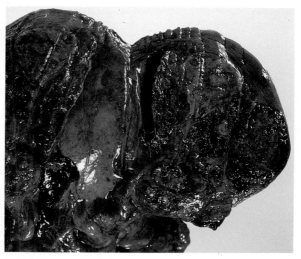

Fig. 8.35

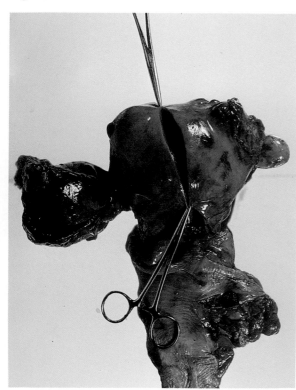

Fig. 8.34

Fig. 8.32 Endometrial hyperplasia. F/45. The patient presented with post-menopausal bleeding. The whole endometrium is involved rather than there being a discrete polyp.

Fig. 8.33 Adenocarcinoma of the endometrium. F/76. There is a large, rather ragged mass of tissue filling the endometrial cavity. It is often difficult to distinguish with certainty between hyperplasia and carcinoma of the endometrium.

Fig. 8.34 Chorioncarcinoma. F/25. Hysterectomy specimen. There is secondary tumour in the right ovary, and the black nodules in the vagina are also secondary tumour.

Fig. 8.35 Cut surface of specimen shown in Fig. 8.34 showing the haemorrhagic tumour invading the myometrium.

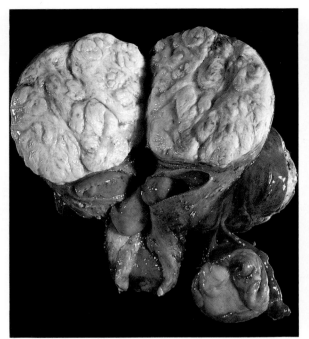

Fig. 8.36

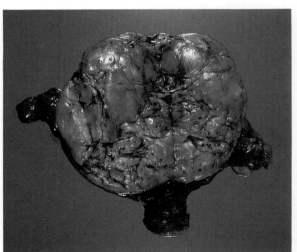

Fig. 8.37

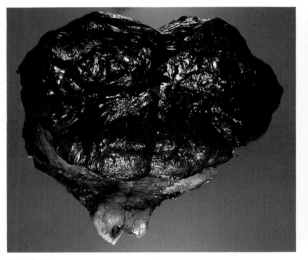

Fig. 8.38

Fig. 8.39

Fig. 8.36 Intra mural leiomyoma. F/40. The typical whorled, lobulated pattern of these tumours is apparent.

Fig. 8.37 Pedunculated leiomyoma protruding through the cervix. F/48.

Fig. 8.38 Red hepatisation in a leiomyoma. F/42. The red, meaty appearance is characteristic.

Fig. 8.39 Lipoleiomyoma. F/45. The yellow appearance of the tumour is due to lipid infiltration.

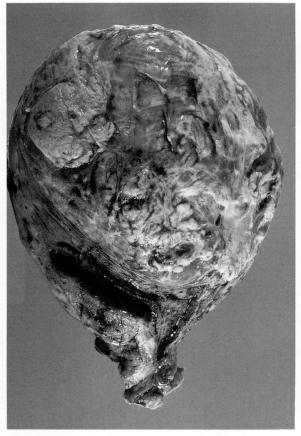

Fig. 8.40

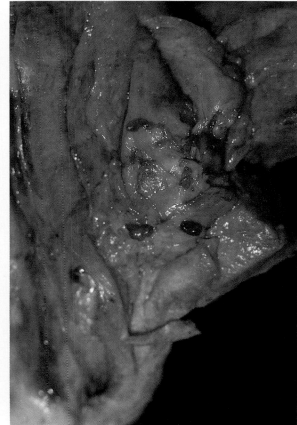

Fig. 8.41

Fig. 8.40 Leiomyoma of the uterus. F/44. The cut surface shows cystic areas and areas of necrosis. This suggested the presence of malignant change, but this was not confirmed on microscopic examination.

Fig. 8.41 Endolymphatic stromal myosis. F/51. Note the red, worm-like areas of tumour in the myometrium.

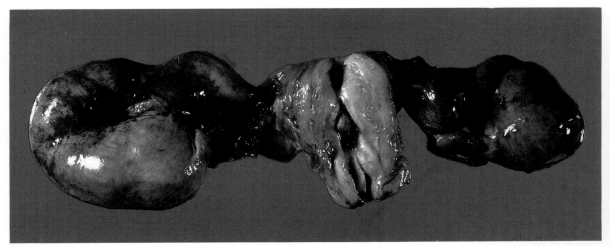

Fig. 8.42

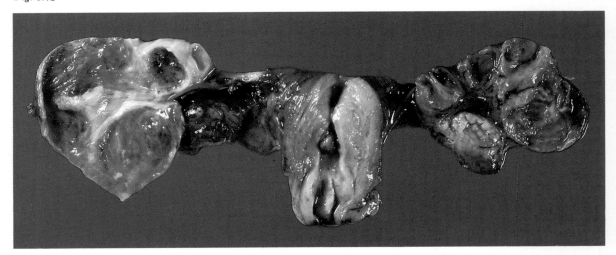

Fig. 8.43

Fig. 8.42 Bilateral pyosalpinx. F/49. The Fallopian tubes are dilated and their serosal surfaces are reddened.

Fig. 8.43 Same specimen as Fig. 8.42. The tubes have been opened to show the pus. A small endometrial polyp is also present.

Fig. 8.44 Hydrosalpinx. F/33. This is an end result of chronic salpingitis. The Fallopian tube is greatly enlarged and filled with clear fluid.

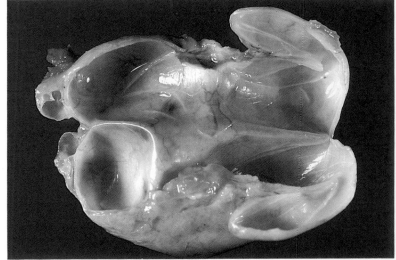

Fig. 8.44

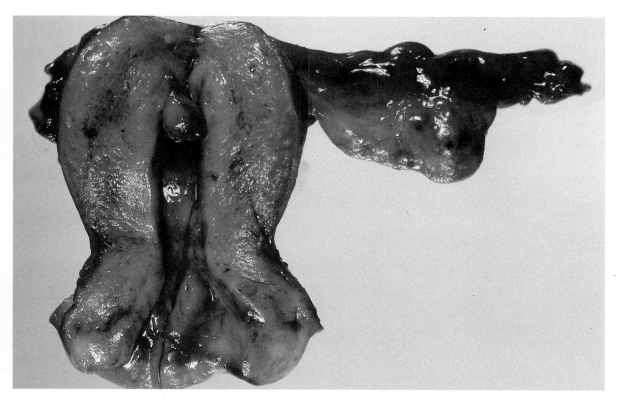

Fig. 8.45

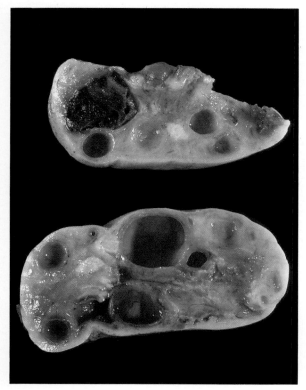

Fig. 8.45 Simple follicular cysts in the ovary. F/40. The unopened cysts have a blue colour.

Fig. 8.46 Bilateral polycystic ovaries. F/23. Most of the cysts are follicular but the one on the left in the upper ovary is a corpus luteum.

Fig. 8.46

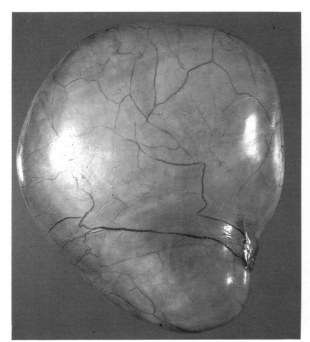

Fig. 8.47

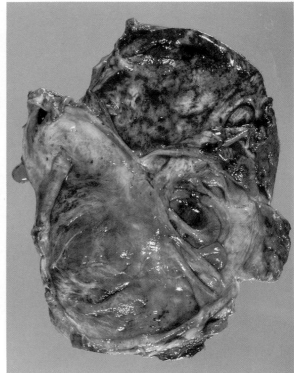

Fig. 8.48

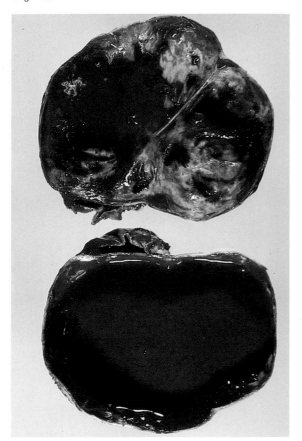

Fig. 8.49

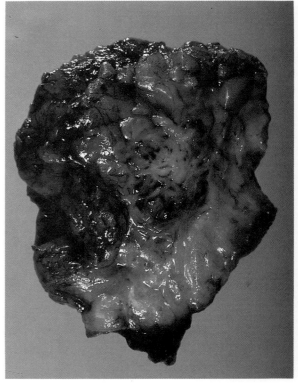

Fig. 8.50

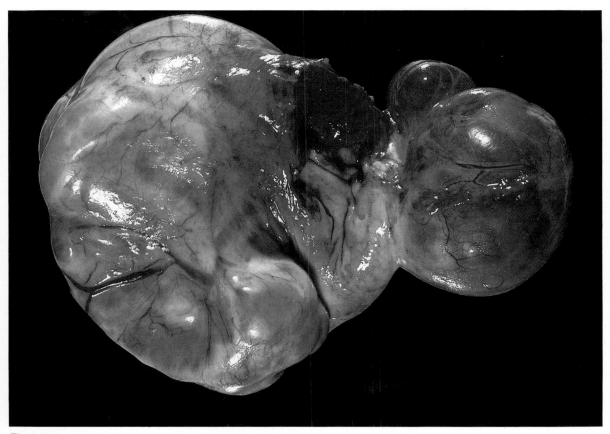

Fig. 8.51

Fig. 8.47 Benign serous cystadenoma of the ovary. F/19. This is a unilocular, thin walled cyst containing clear fluid.

Fig. 8.48 Endometriosis of the ovary. F/40. The ovarian cyst is multiloculated. The blood has been removed from most of the loculi.

Fig. 8.49 Endometriosis of the ovary. F/31. Blood has not been removed so as to demonstrate the so-called 'chocolate cyst'.

Fig. 8.50 Extra pelvic endometriosis. F/43. A subcutaneous lump appeared at the site of an abdominal scar, the result of Caesarian section five years previously. This was excised, and on cross-section the blood-filled cysts can be seen in the centre of the specimen.

Fig. 8.51 Benign mucinous cystadenoma of the ovary. F/76. The solid tumour on the left is a benign Brenner tumour. This combination is quite frequent.

Fig. 8.52 The cut surface shows a multiloculated cyst containing mucin, most of which has been removed. F/64.

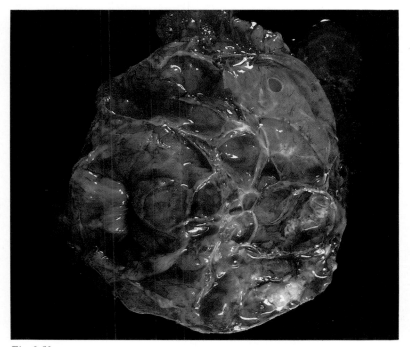

Fig. 8.52

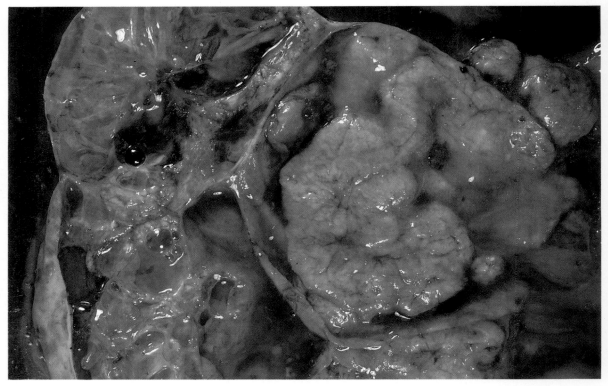

Fig. 8.53

Fig. 8.53 Mucinous cystadenocarcinoma of the ovary. F/47. Solid areas of tumour are present as well as multiple loculi of benign mucinous cystadenoma.

Fig. 8.54 Papillary cystadenocarcinoma of the ovary. F/32. Note the papillary projections in the lumen of the cyst and also on its surface. In a benign papillary cystadenoma the papillae are present only on the inner surface of the cyst.

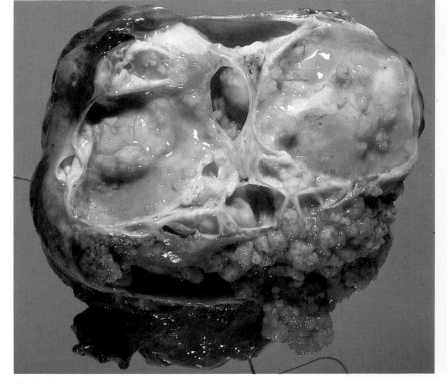

Fig. 8.54

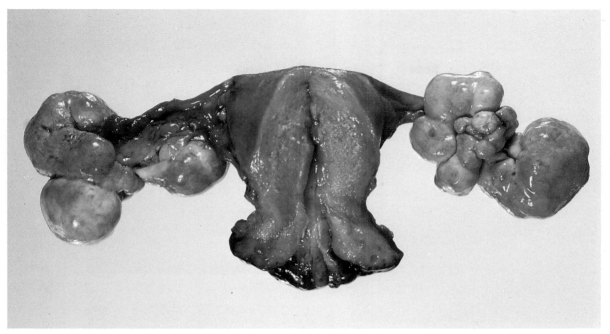

Fig. 8.55

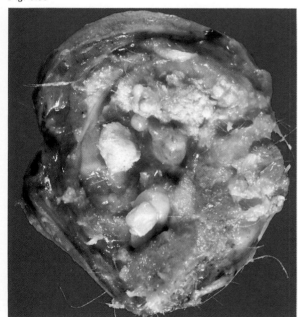

Fig. 8.56

Fig. 8.55 Krukenberg tumour. F/44. Both ovaries are fairly symmetrically enlarged and replaced by secondary adenocarcinoma.

Fig. 8.56 Dermoid cyst (benign teratoma) of the ovary. F/26. It contains sebaceous material, hair and a tooth.

Fig. 8.57 Torsion of an ovarian Dermoid cyst and the attached Fallopian tube. F/23.

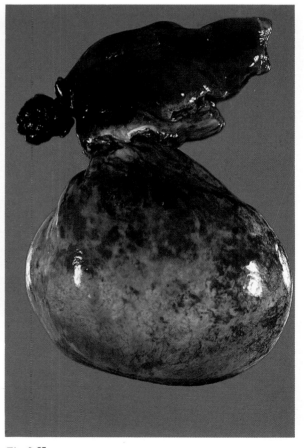

Fig. 8.57

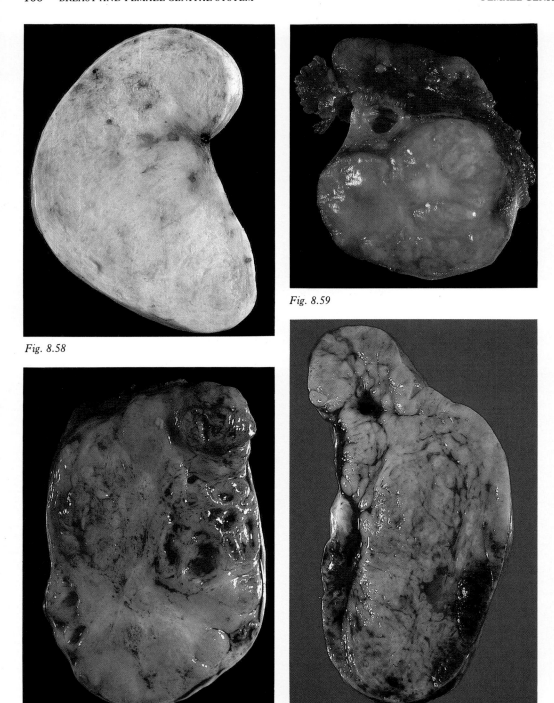

Fig. 8.58

Fig. 8.59

Fig. 8.60

Fig. 8.61

Fig. 8.58 Fibroma of the ovary. F/30. The cut surface of the tumour shows a homogeneous white appearance.

Fig. 8.59 Thecoma of the ovary. F/66. It is distinguished from fibroma by the presence of lipid which gives it a yellow colour.

Fig. 8.60 Granulosa cell tumour of the ovary. F/84. These tumours, too, are usually yellow. Positive diagnosis depends on the microscopic appearances. They sometimes secrete oestrogen.

Fig. 8.61 Dysgerminoma of the ovary. F/30. The tumour has a cream coloured, fleshy appearance on its cut surface.

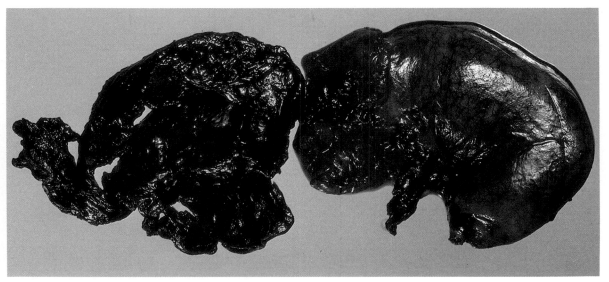

Fig. 8.62

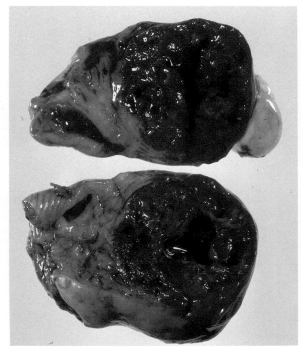

Fig. 8.63

Fig. 8.62 Ruptured tubal ectopic pregnancy. F/24. Blood and placental tissue is exuding from the greatly distended Fallopian tube.

Fig. 8.63 Ovarian pregnancy. F/32. The placental tissue is embedded in the ovary.

Fig. 8.64 Lithopaedion. F/55. This was removed from the pelvic wall. It was an incidental finding during pelvic surgery.

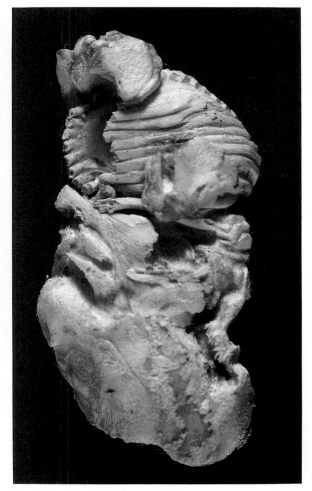

Fig. 8.64

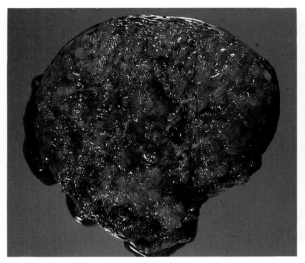

Fig. 8.65

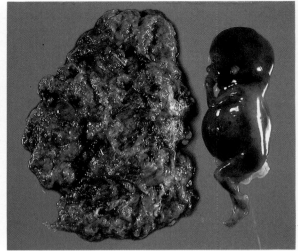

Fig. 8.66

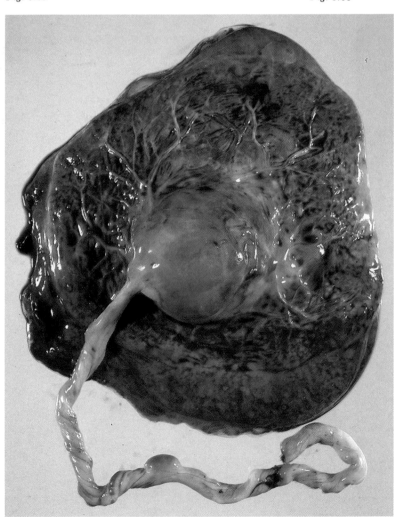

Fig. 8.67

Fig. 8.65 Hydatidiform mole. F/29. Hysterectomy specimen. Note the variably sized vesicles, no normal placenta and no fetus.

Fig. 8.66 Partial mole. F/30. Note the presence of normal placenta plus some variably sized vesicles. The fetus is abnormal, and chromosomal studies showed it to be triploid—69, XXX.

Fig. 8.67 Chorangioma (benign haemangioma) of the placenta. This tumour usually occurs at the site of insertion of the cord and is the commonest tumour of the placenta.

Fig. 8.68 Placenta with retroplacental haemorrhage.

Fig. 8.69 Placenta with broad, depressed areas of infarction.

Fig. 8.70 Erythroblastosis foetalis. Large oedematous placenta.

Fig. 8.71 Large oedematous stillborn fetus (Hydrops fetalis from Rhesus incompatibility).

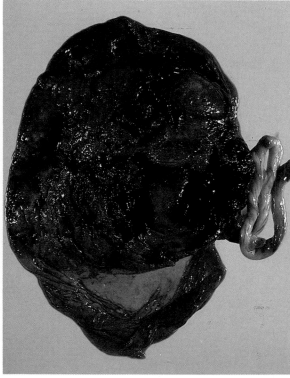

Fig. 8.68

Fig. 8.69

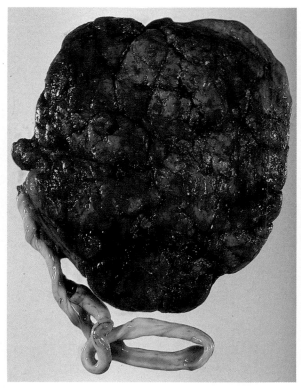

Fig. 8.70

Fig. 8.71

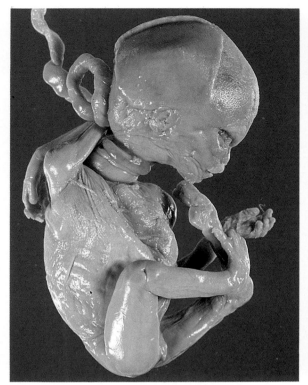

Fig. 8.72

Fig. 8.73

Fig. 8.72 Knotting of the umbilical cord around the neck of the fetus. This resulted in intrauterine death.

Fig. 8.73 Intrauterine Candidiasis. White spots of Candida colonies are present on the surface of the umbilical cord.

Fig. 8.74 Placenta accreta. F/30. Hysterectomy was performed to stop the post-partum haemorrhage when the placenta could not be removed manually after delivery of the baby.

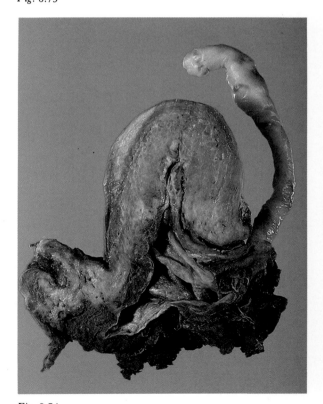

Fig. 8.74

9

Endocrine system

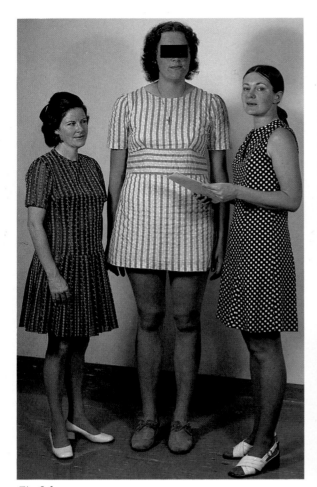

Fig. 9.1

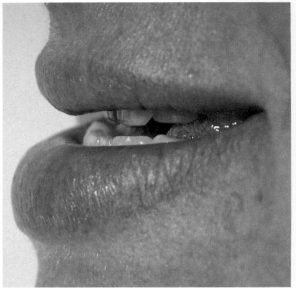

Fig. 9.2

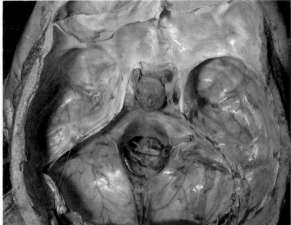

Fig. 9.4

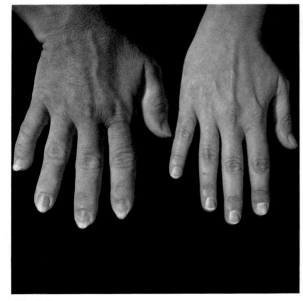

Fig. 9.3

Fig. 9.1 Hyperpituitarism. Gigantism. F/19. Family photographs showed that this young woman had consistently outgrown her twin brother and was always the biggest child in the school class. She had a pituitary adenoma secreting growth hormone.

Fig. 9.2 Acromegaly. F/36. The photograph shows the characteristic malocclusion of the teeth resulting from the overgrowth of the mandible. The patient had noticed that over the past few years her facial appearance had been changing.

Fig. 9.3 Acromegaly. The enlarged, spade-shaped hand of the patient in Fig. 9.2 is shown on the left with a normal for comparison.

Fig. 9.4 Pituitary adenoma in situ. There is extension of the tumour anteriorly, compressing the right optic nerve. The majority of pituitary adenomas are chromophobe tumours tinctorially. Some cause symptoms because of their compression of adjacent structures, while others do so because of their secretion of hormones.

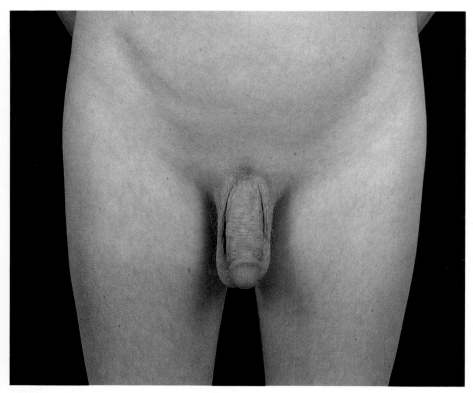

Fig. 9.5

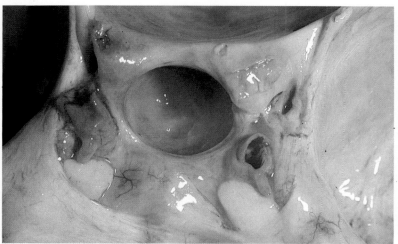

Fig. 9.6

Fig. 9.7

Fig. 9.5 Hypopituitarism. Hypogonadism. M/20. There are many causes for this, one of which is pituitary failure.

Fig. 9.6 Hypopituitarism. M/64. At the post mortem on this patient, the pituitary fossa was empty and no pituitary tissue could be found.

Fig. 9.7 Cystic pituitary gland. F/55. The patient had had hypopituitarism since the birth of her last child which was associated with heavy post-partum bleeding. Presumably, this caused infarction of the pituitary—Sheehan's Syndrome.

Fig. 9.8 Cushing's Syndrome. F/45. Over a period of approximately two years this woman had noticed increasing obesity associated with a round face and red cheeks.

Fig. 9.9 The same patient as in Fig. 9.8 showing truncal obesity and livid striae.

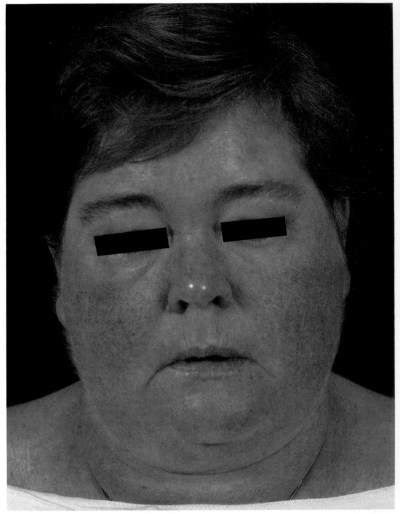

Fig. 9.8

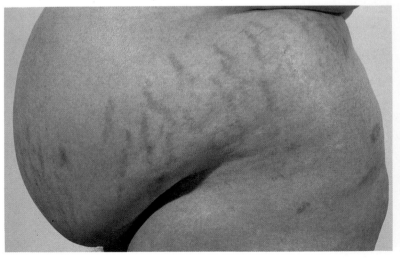

Fig. 9.9

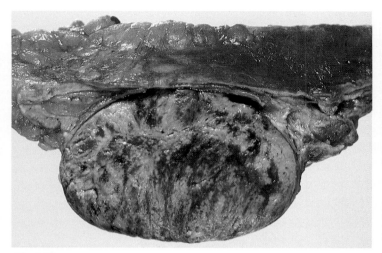

Fig. 9.10

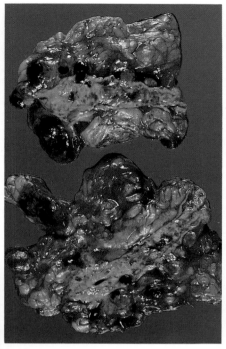

Fig. 9.12

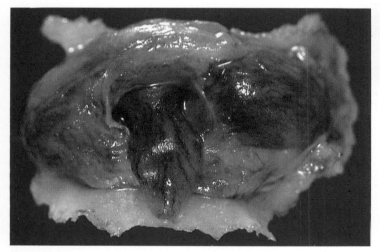

Fig. 9.11

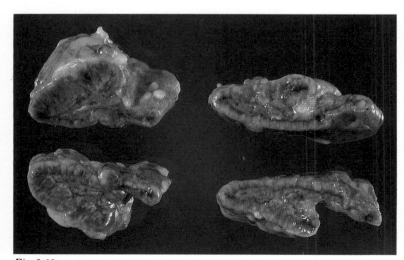

Fig. 9.13

Fig. 9.10 Cushing's Syndrome.
Adrenal cortical adenoma. F/29. This
tumour was removed surgically.

Fig. 9.11 Basophil adenoma of the
pituitary. F/66. This patient died with
Cushing's Syndrome and the basophil
adenoma was found at post mortem.

Fig. 9.12 Bilateral focal nodular
hyperplasia of the adrenal. F/31. This
patient had Cushing's Syndrome and
the left adrenal gland was removed.
When this failed to control the
Cushing's, a right adrenalectomy was
performed. The periadrenal fat was
removed with the gland to ensure that
the nodules of adrenal tissue which
extended into it were completely
removed.

Fig. 9.13 Bilateral adrenal hyperplasia.
F/66. The adrenals from the patient in
Fig. 9.11. Both adrenals are markedly
enlarged and are a brown colour because
the hyperplasia occurs mainly in the
zona reticularis. Adrenal hyperplasia
such as this may be primary, in which
case it is a cause of Cushing's
Syndrome. Or it may be secondary to
endogenous secretion or exogenous
administration of ACTH.

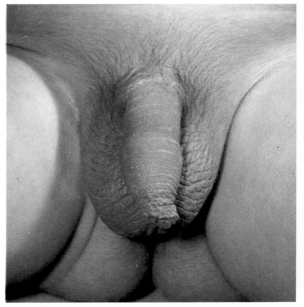

Fig. 9.14

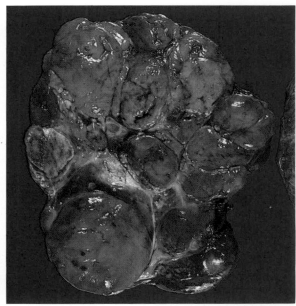

Fig. 9.15

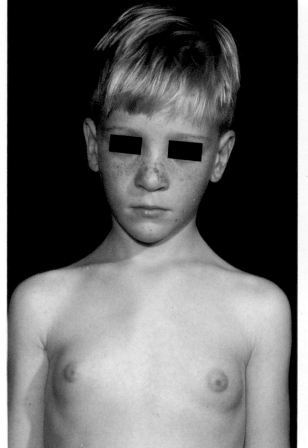

Fig. 9.16

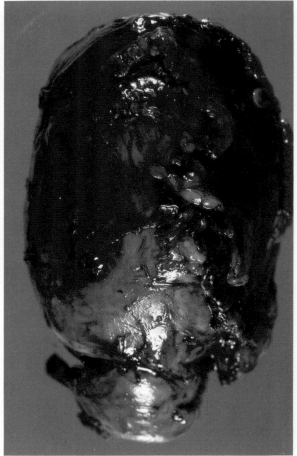

Fig. 9.17

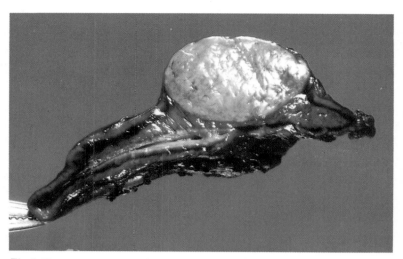

Fig. 9.18

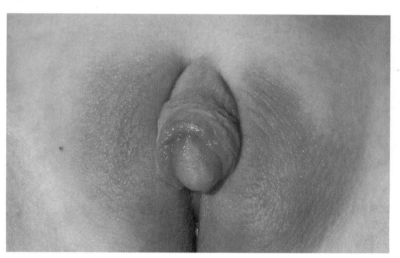

Fig. 9.19

Fig. 9.14 Precocious puberty. M/11 months.

Fig. 9.15 Adrenal cortical adenoma. This was removed surgically from the patient in Fig. 9.14. The cut surface is multilobulated and a homogeneous brown colour. This adenoma was secreting androgens.

Fig. 9.16 Gynaecomastia. M/5.

Fig. 9.17 Adrenal cortical tumour. This large adrenal tumour was removed surgically from the patient in Fig. 9.16. It was secreting oestrogens. The tumour was somewhat adherent to adjacent structures and was torn during removal. It is impossible to predict which adrenal tumours will be malignant, because cellular pleomorphism does not correlate with their behaviour. In spite of the local adhesions and raggedness of this specimen, the gynaecomastia subsided and the patient was alive and well ten years post-operatively.

Fig. 9.18 Conn's Syndrome. M/58. Surgical specimen of the left adrenal gland showing a bright yellow cortical adenoma. The patient presented with hypertension and hypokalaemia. Both of these were reversed by the adrenalectomy.

Fig. 9.19 Adreno-genital Syndrome. F/2½. These patients have pseudohermaphrodite genitalia because of hypertrophy of the clitoris. The condition is caused by enzyme deficiency in the adrenal gland resulting in over production of androgens.

Fig. 9.20 Addison's Disease. M/40. This man presented with heavy pigmentation of the skin and blotchy pigmentation of the tongue.

Fig. 9.21 On the right is the hand of the patient in Fig. 9.20 showing increased pigmentation, particularly in the palmar creases, and on the left is a normal hand for comparison.

Fig. 9.22 Adrenal atrophy in Addison's Disease. The diseased atrophic adrenal is compared with a normal one.

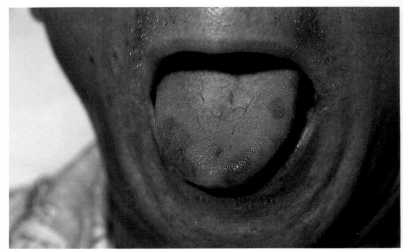

Fig. 9.20

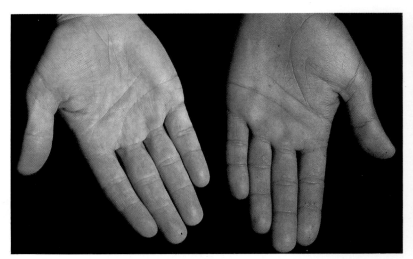

Fig. 9.21

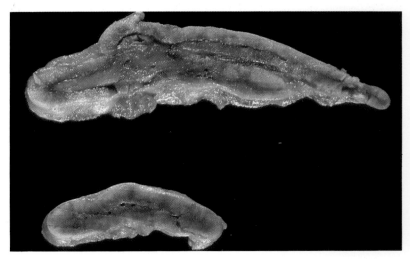

Fig. 9.22

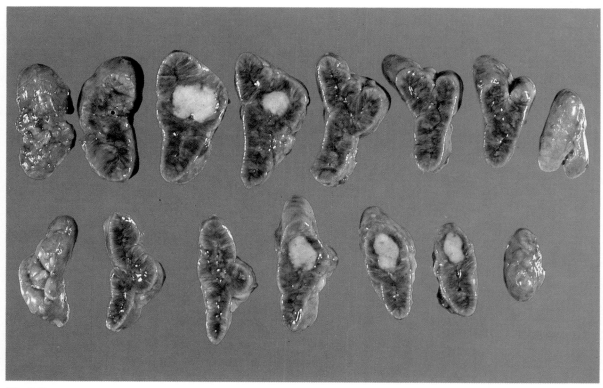

Fig. 9.23

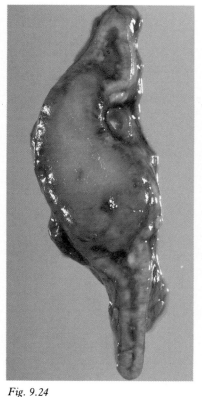

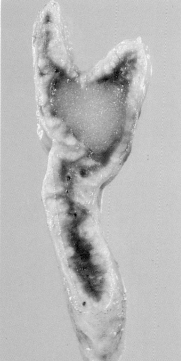

Fig. 9.23 Bilateral adrenal hyperplasia caused by an oat cell carcinoma of the lung. M/56. Both adrenals have been sliced to show that they are enlarged and brown. There are secondary deposits from the lung cancer in the medulla of both adrenals. Towards the end of his life, the patient had clinical features of Cushing's Syndrome. This is an example of hormone secretion by a non-endocrine tumour.

Fig. 9.24 Secondary lung cancer in the medulla of the adrenal. M/51. Sometimes secondary tumour completely replaces both adrenals, and the patient suffers from Addison's Disease in the last few weeks of life.

Fig. 9.25 Myelolipoma in the medulla of the adrenal. F/84. An incidental post mortem finding.

Fig. 9.24   *Fig. 9.25*

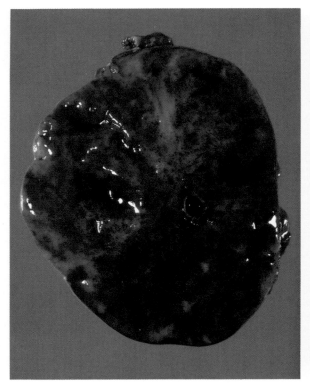

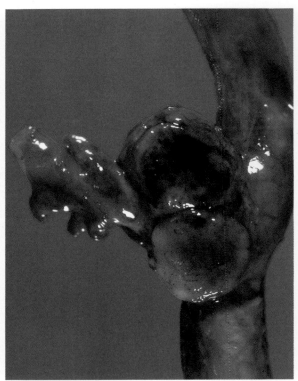

Fig. 9.26

Fig. 9.27

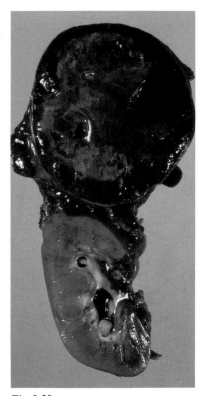

Fig. 9.26 Phaeochromocytoma almost completely replacing the left adrenal gland. F/35. The patient presented with hypertension which was cured by removal of the tumour. The cut surface of the tumour shows a red, haemorrhagic appearance. There is a tiny remnant of adrenal cortex at the top of the specimen.

Fig. 9.27 Carotid body tumour. F/80. This tumour is an example of a chemodectoma. This particular one was an incidental post mortem finding.

Fig. 9.28 Neuroblastoma. M/4½. The haemorrhagic tumour has replaced the right adrenal gland. The child presented with a mass in the right upper quadrant of the abdomen and it was surgically removed. This treatment formed part of the combined surgical, radiotherapy and chemotherapeutic treatment.

Fig. 9.29   Hyperparathyroidism. M/51. Three glands were removed at parathyroidectomy and laid out in accordance with their anatomical distribution. The right upper gland is very large and weighed 3.8 g. The right lower is a biopsy, and the left lower is a little larger than normal. The patient presented with asymptomatic hypercalcaemia. The calcium returned to normal post-operatively and remained normal. Terminology in this condition is somewhat difficult. 'What constitutes an adenoma and what constitutes hyperplasia'. This one could be regarded as being one large and one small adenoma.

Fig. 9.30 Hyperparathyroid bone disease. F/72. The segment of vertebral column shows bands of dense bone on each side of the intervertebral discs. This has been called the 'rugger jersy' spine and is seen particularly in secondary hyperparathyroidism.

Fig. 9.31 Secondary hyperparathyroidism. M/40. All four parathyroid glands are very markedly enlarged. The patient had chronic renal disease and the hyperplastic parathyroids were becoming autonomous and were removed. The surgeon left a small piece of one parathyroid gland in situ in order to preserve some parathyroid function.

Fig. 9.32 The cut surfaces of the parathyroids in Fig. 9.31. This shows the multilobulated appearance of the hyperplastic parathyroid glands.

Fig. 9.28

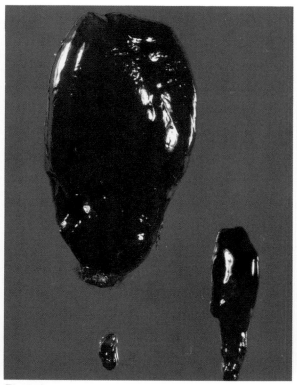

Fig. 9.29

Fig. 9.30

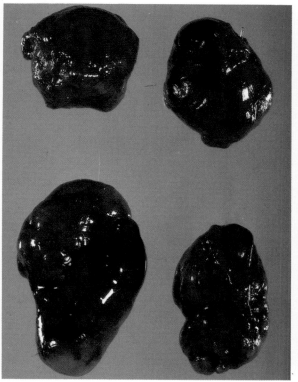

Fig. 9.31

Fig. 9.32

Fig. 9.33 Large goitre. F/45.

Fig. 9.34 Multinodular colloid goitre
The cut surface of the gland is
multilobulated and the lobules vary in
size. Glistening colloid can be seen on
the cut surface.

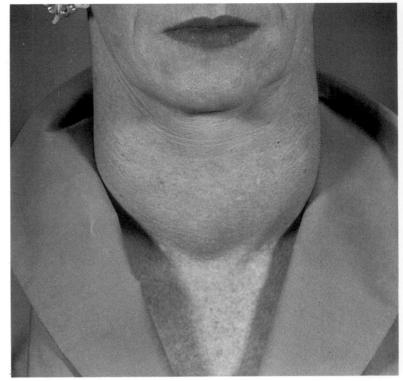

Fig. 9.33

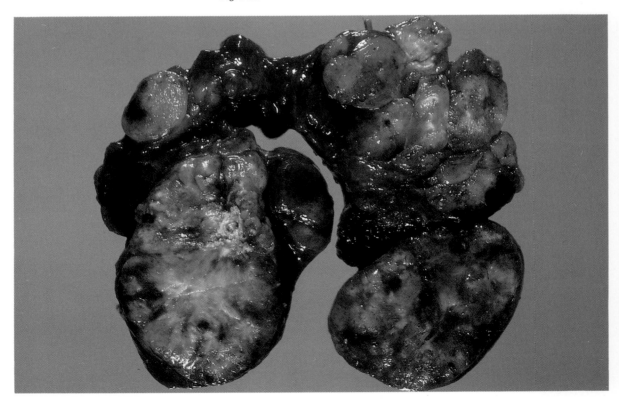

Fig. 9.34

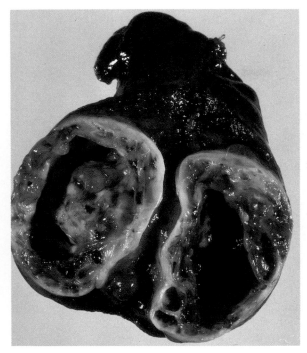

Fig. 9.35

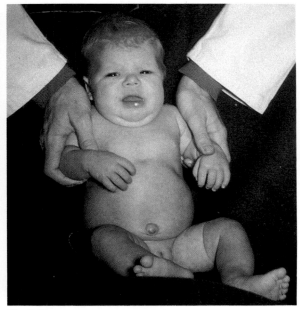

Fig. 9.36

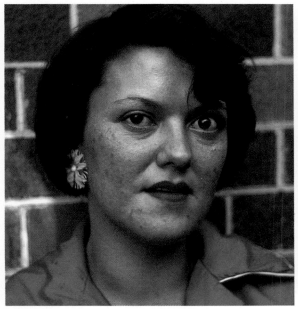

Fig. 9.37

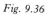
Fig. 9.38

Fig. 9.35 Thyroid cyst. F/46. This presented as a unilateral enlargement of thyroid. It was hard on palpation because of calcification in its wall.

Fig. 9.36 Follicular adenoma of thyroid. F/35. This presented as a solitary enlargement of one lateral lobe of the thyroid. The cut surface shows a single well circumscribed nodule of brownish coloured tissue.

Fig. 9.37 Thyrotoxicosis. F/26. Note the presence of the smooth symmetrical goitre and a minor degree of exophthalmos. It is now rare to see surgical specimens of untreated thyrotoxicosis, because medical treatment is always tried first.

Fig. 9.38 Cretin. F/4 months. The baby had a hoarse cry, was floppy, could not sit up and the hair was coarse and reddish.

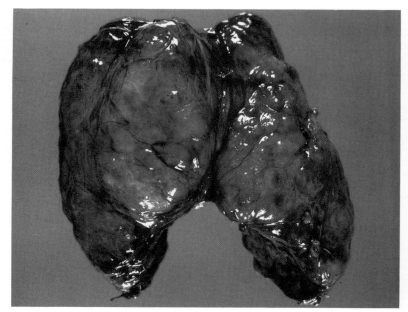

Fig. 9.39

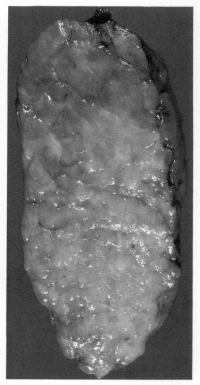

Fig. 9.40

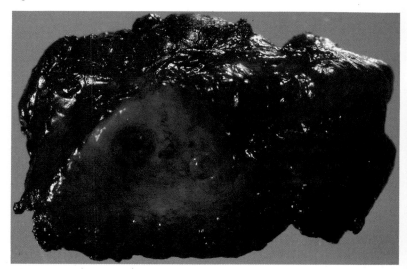

Fig. 9.41

Fig. 9.39 Hashimoto's Thyroiditis. F/45. Subtotal thyroidectomy of a moderately enlarged thyroid gland.

Fig. 9.40 Cut surface of the gland from Fig. 9.39. It shows the nodular, fleshy appearance, characteristic of this condition. No colloid can be seen.

Fig. 9.41 Granulomatous thyroiditis. F/60. This lady presented with a unilateral thyroid enlargement. There is a firm, homogeneous area in the middle of the specimen. Microscopic sections showed granulomatous thyroiditis.

Fig. 9.42 Riedel's Thyroiditis. F/60. The abnormal thyroid was an unexpected post mortem finding. The gland was hard and woody and was firmly attached to the strap muscles of the neck.

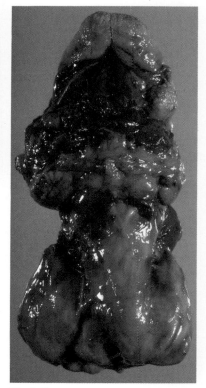

Fig. 9.42

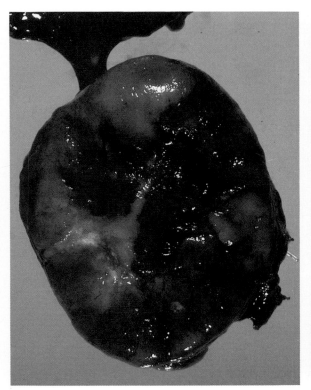

Fig. 9.43

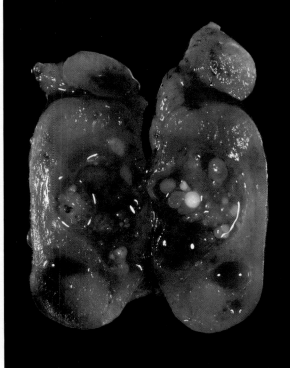

Fig. 9.44

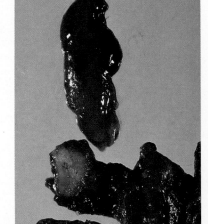

Fig. 9.45

Fig. 9.46

Fig. 9.43 Follicular carcinoma of the thyroid. F/46. The patient presented with unilateral enlargement of the thyroid and a single thyroid nodule was removed. It appears to be well circumscribed with a fairly homogeneous cut surface. The diagnosis of follicular carcinoma depends on the microscopic demonstration of vessel invasion, or the presence of metastases.

Fig. 9.44 Secondary papillary carcinoma of the thyroid in a cervical lymph node. F/25. This patient presented with cervical lymphadenopathy. One of the nodes was removed and when it was cut across, a focus of colloid-containing thyroid tissue was visible.

Fig. 9.45 Multifocal papillary carcinoma of the thyroid. F/21. Tumour is present throughout the enlarged gland.

Fig. 9.46 Solitary papillary carcinoma of the thyroid. F/29. This tumour occurs in the ways demonstrated in Figs. 9.44 and 9.45 but sometimes, when secondaries are present in cervical lymph nodes, it is almost impossible to find a primary tumour in the thyroid gland itself.

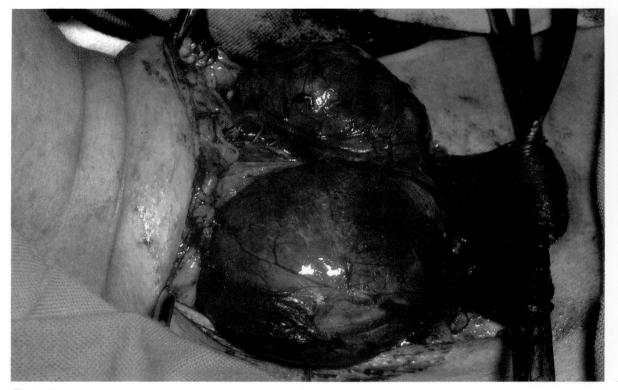

Fig. 9.47

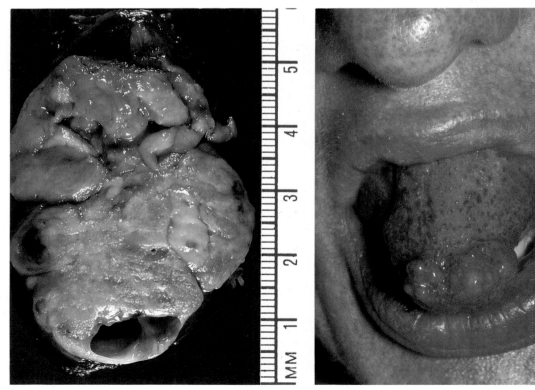

Fig. 9.48

Fig. 9.49

Fig. 9.47 Medullary carcinoma of the thyroid. F/40. Tumour involved both lobes of the gland, causing considerable enlargement, as shown in this operative photograph.

Fig. 9.48 Medullary carcinoma of the thyroid. Cut surface of the tumour from Fig. 9.47. It is fleshy and yellowish in colour.

Fig. 9.49 Multiple adenomata on the tip of the tongue of the patient in Fig. 9.47.

Fig. 9.50 Phaeochromocytoma. One of the bilateral phaeochromocytomas removed from the patient in Fig. 9.47. The tumour has a reddish, homogeneous appearance with a cystic area in the middle. Normal adrenal tissue can be seen on the bottom right and the top left of the specimen. The patient's sister had similar pathology. They were both suffering from one of the varieties of the **multiple endocrine adenopathy syndrome**—type 2B.

Fig. 9.51 Secondary medullary carcinoma of the thyroid in the liver. F/55. This lady had a medullary carcinoma of the thyroid removed 21 years before she presented with Cushing's Syndrome, three months before her death. This demonstrates two of the other features of medullary carcinoma. One, that it grows slowly and metastases may not appear until many years after removal of the primary. Two, it is one of the tumours that produces ACTH and the clinical presentation may occur because of the effects of this.

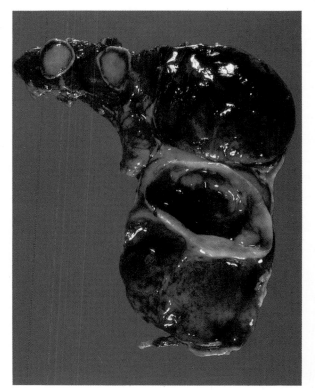

Fig. 9.50

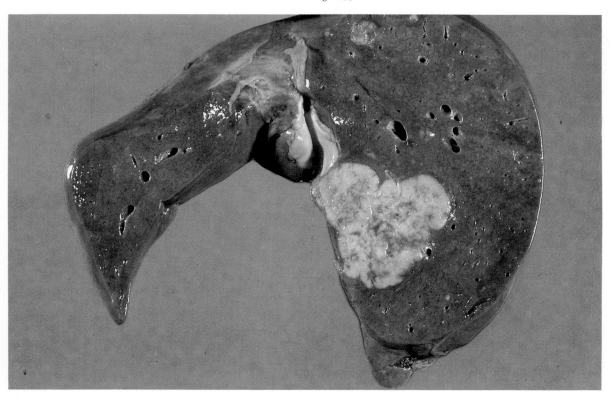

Fig. 9.51

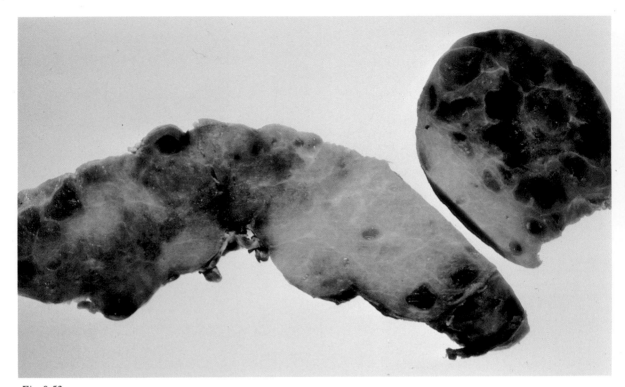

Fig. 9.52

Fig. 9.54

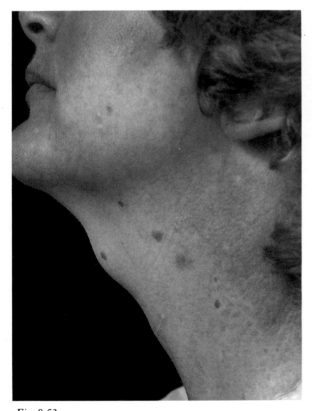

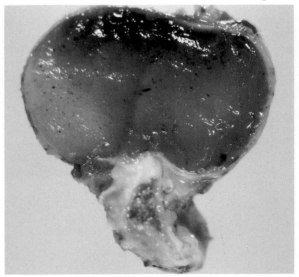

Fig. 9.52 Amyloid goitre. F/12 from Papua New Guinea. The thyroid has been almost completely replaced by firm, homogeneous pale tissue which microscopically was amyloid. Amyloid goitre is relatively common in Papua New Guinea.

Fig. 9.53 Thyroglossal cyst. F/40. Situated in the midline, just above the thyroid cartilage.

Fig. 9.54 Thyroglossal cyst. Surgical specimen showing the cyst filled with glistening colloid.

Fig. 9.53

10

Bones, joints and connective tissue

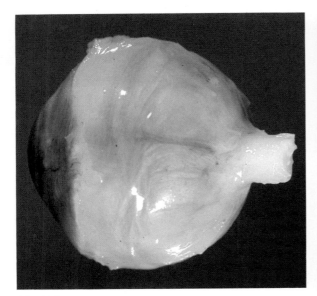

Fig. 10.1

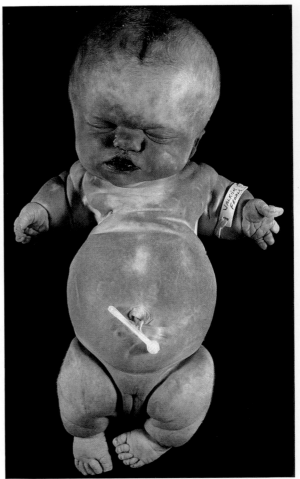

Fig. 10.2

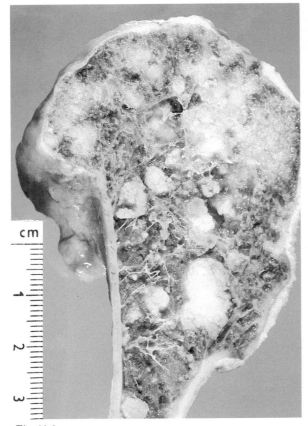

Fig. 10.3

Fig. 10.1 Osteogenesis imperfecta. Patients with this condition have abnormally fragile bones and suffer multiple repeated fractures. They usually have blue coloured sclerotics as is shown in this eye from a child who died from this condition.

Fig. 10.2 Achondroplasia. This stillborn fetus demonstrates the short arms and legs of this inherited abnormality of endochondral ossification. People with this condition may be seen as dwarfs in circuses and theatre productions.

Fig. 10.3 Multiple enchondromata (Ollier's Disease). M/28. The head of the humerus is greatly expanded by the intramedullary chondromas.

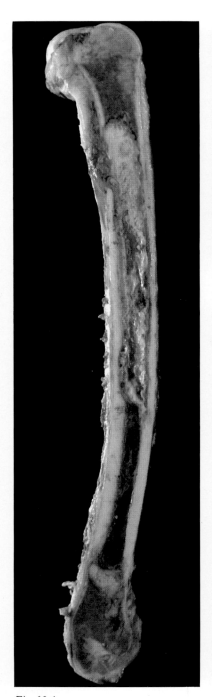

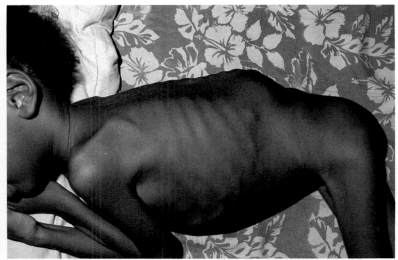

Fig. 10.5

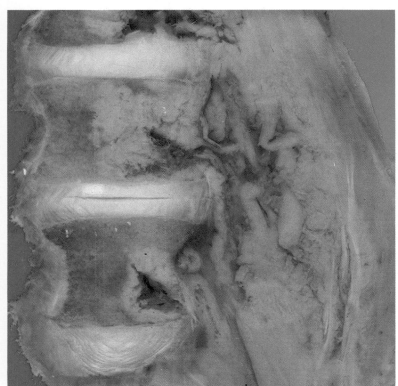

Fig. 10.4   Fig. 10.6

Fig. 10.4 Osteomyelitis. F/21. There is a large collection of pus in the medullary cavity of the shaft of the femur. This patient died from acute leukaemia and the infection resulted from her immune deficiency state.

Fig. 10.5 Tuberculosis of the spine. F/4. This child from Papua New Guinea is grossly emaciated from the disseminated infection, and the deformity in the lumbar region is

characteristic of involvement of the lumbar vertebrae by tuberculous infection.

Fig. 10.6 Tuberculous psoas abscess. Two lumbar vertebrae involved by tuberculosis with extension of the caseation into the psoas muscle. When such infection spreads along the psoas, the abscess may 'point' in the groin.

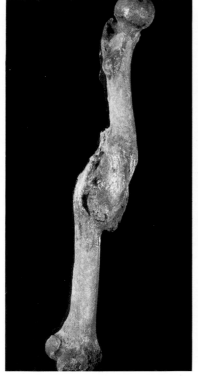
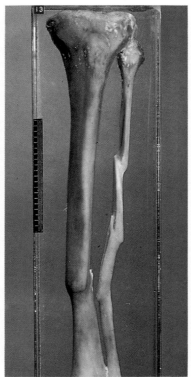
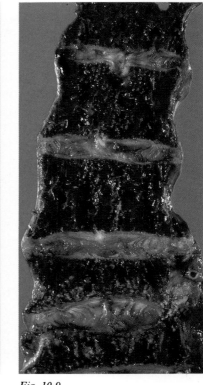

Fig. 10.7   *Fig. 10.8*   *Fig. 10.9*

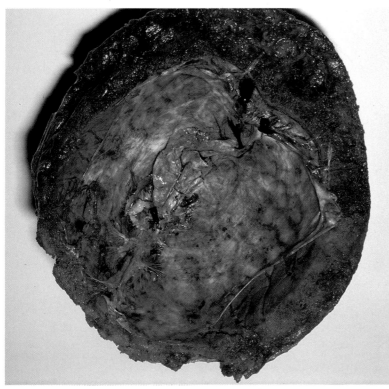
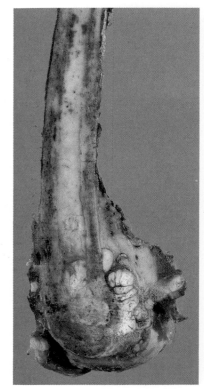

Fig. 10.10   *Fig. 10.11*

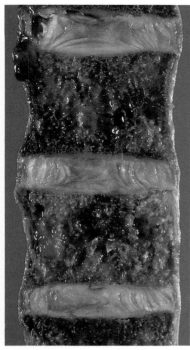

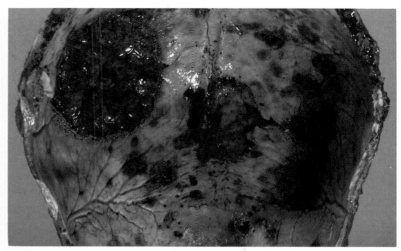

Fig. 10.13

Fig. 10.12

Fig. 10.7 Healed fracture. Femur recovered by archaeologists from a burial about 2000 years ago. There has been a fracture which has healed with a great deal of callus formation.

Fig. 10.8 Multiple fractures of the tibia and fibula which have healed with very little callus—a tribute to modern splinting methods for the treatment of fractures.

Fig. 10.9 Osteoporosis. F/65. The trabecular bone in the vertebral bodies is very thin and the two lower vertebrae show the effects of crush fracture—a complication of this condition.

Fig. 10.10 Paget's Disease of the skull. F/81. Note the gross thickening of the diploe of the skull. The bone is extremely vascular.

Fig. 10.11 Paget's Disease with osteogenic sarcoma. M/64. The sliced femur shows thickening of the cortical bone which is abnormally vascular and abnormally soft. Bowing of long bones is often seen and fractures are frequent. An osteogenic sarcoma has developed at the lower end of the femur. This is a well known complication.

Fig. 10.12 Secondary carcinoma in the lumbar vertebrae. M/68. Cream coloured homogeneous deposits can be seen in each vertebral body, the biggest being in the lower one. The primary tumour was a bronchogenic carcinoma of the lung.

Fig. 10.13 Skull in multiple myeloma. M/39. Multiple, rounded, red deposits of myeloma are present in the calvarium. These are seen as round holes on skull X-ray.

Fig. 10.14 Vertebral column in multiple myeloma. The same patient as in Fig. 10.12. The myeloma deposits in the vertebrae cause loss of bone and consequent crush fractures as demonstrated here.

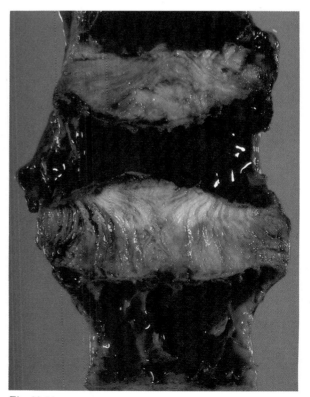

Fig. 10.14

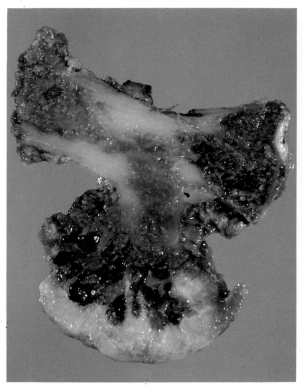

Fig. 10.15

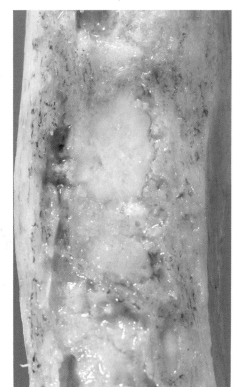

Fig. 10.16

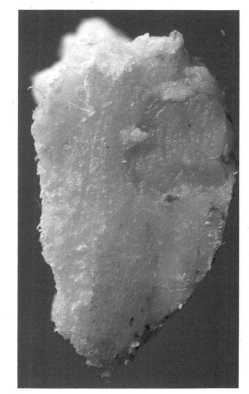

Fig. 10.17

Fig. 10.18

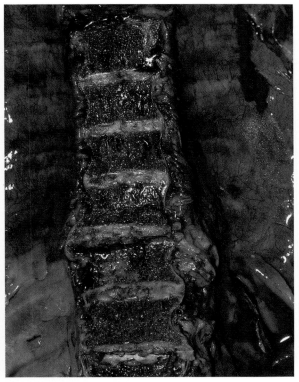

Fig. 10.19

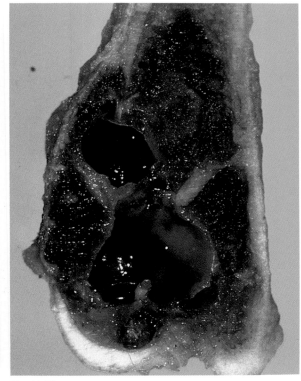

Fig. 10.20

Fig. 10.15 Osteochondroma on a rib.
F/22. This is a common benign tumour which usually occurs in the region of the epiphyses of long bones. It is characterised by having a distinct cartilage cap. Such tumours are easily excised.

Fig. 10.16 Osteoid osteoma in the proximal phalanx of a finger. M/30. There is a benign, well circumscribed tumour within the medullary cavity. The treatment of choice is local curettage. Amputation such as this is over treatment.

Fig. 10.17 Benign chondroma. M/27. This small cartilage tumour was resected from the tibia.

Fig. 10.18 Fibrous dysplasia in the medullary cavity of the midshaft of the tibia. F/14.

Fig. 10.19 Multiple benign haemangiomas in the vertebrae. F/68. This was an incidental post mortem finding. Haemangiomas of bone may be single or multiple.

Fig. 10.20 Aneurysmal bone cyst in the lower end of the ulna. M/40. The large angiomatous spaces are expanding the cortex of the bone.

Fig. 10.21 Osteogenic sarcoma. F/11. The creamy tumour has involved the lower end of the femur and has broken through the cortical bone and caused elevation of the periosteum.

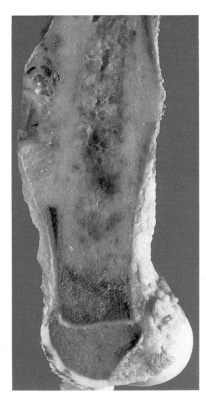

Fig. 10.21

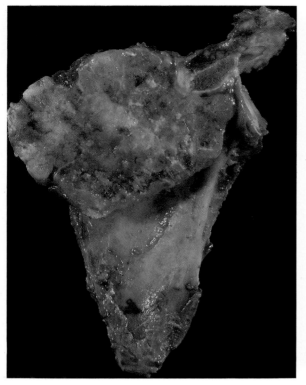

Fig. 10.22

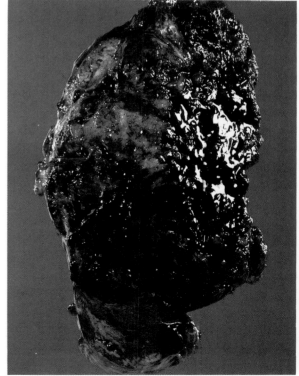

Fig. 10.23

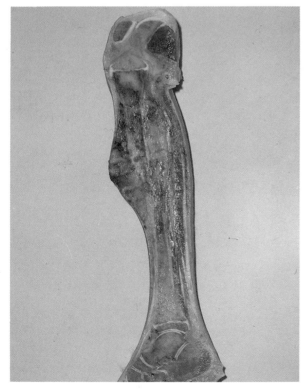

Fig. 10.24

Fig. 10.25

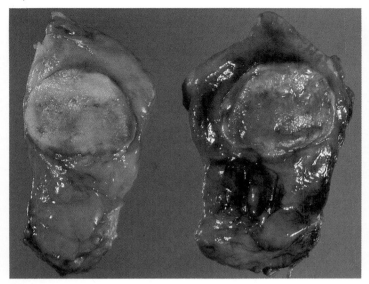

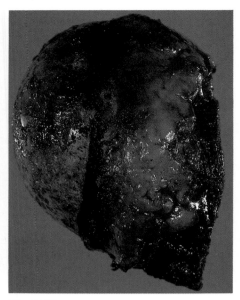

Fig. 10.26

Fig. 10.27

Fig. 10.22 Chondrosarcoma arising in the scapula. F/35. This tumour had grown rapidly. Its cut surface shows a lobulated pattern with the white, glistening appearance of cartilage.

Fig. 10.23 Giant cell tumour in the upper end of the femur. F/42. The haemorrhagic areas of tumour are easily visible. This is in fact a recurrence of a tumour which was treated by curettage, as shown by the paucity of trabecular bone in the upper end of the femur. The bone was stabilised by insertion of a nail at the time of the original operation. The nail track is clearly visible. When recurrence of tumour occurred in the greater trochanter and in the neck of the femur, amputation was performed.

Fig. 10.24 Ewing's tumour. M/13. A large tumour in the upper third of the tibia has eroded the cortical bone and has extended beneath the periosteum. There is a pathological fracture through the tumour.

Fig. 10.25 Chordoma removed from the pelvis anterior to the sacrum. M/58. The tumour is haemorrhagic and has a rather mucoid cut surface. Microscopic examination was required to make a definitive diagnosis.

Fig. 10.26 Chronic osteoarthritis. F/67. Both patellae have been removed. They show irregular eburnation of their articular surfaces.

Fig. 10.27 Osteoarthritis and ochronosis. M/58. The head of the femur was amputated during an operation for insertion of an artificial hip joint. The patient had had painful, osteoarthritic hips for some years. The specimen shows overgrowth of bone with the formation of osteophytes along the line of the resection, and irregularity of the articular cartilage. These are features of osteoarthritis and the only special feature is the wide band of black pigment running across the articular cartilage. Ochronosis is characterised by melanin pigmentation of articular cartilage. Patients with this abnormality are particularly prone to develop osteoarthritis.

Fig. 10.28 Ochronosis. The right eye of the patient from Fig. 10.27 shows deposition of melanin in the sclerotic.

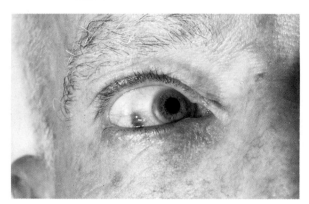

Fig. 10.28

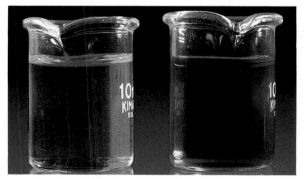

Fig. 10.29

Fig. 10.29 Urine from the same patient. The sample on the left is freshly voided, and that on the right has been standing for two hours, during which time it has turned dark brown. Figs. 10.27–10.29 illustrate the cardinal features of the hereditary metabolic disease, Alcaptonuria.

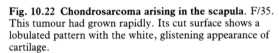

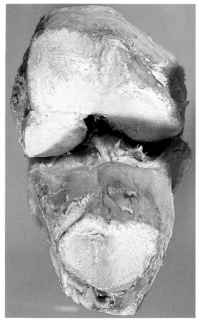

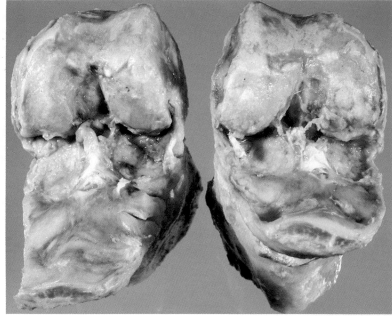

Fig. 10.30

Fig. 10.31

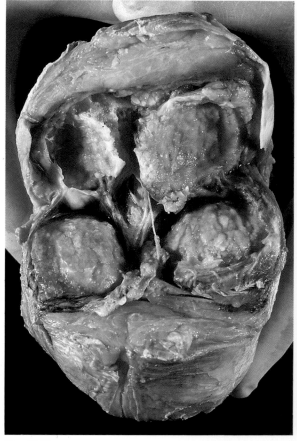

Fig. 10.30 Knee joint in gout. M/76. The knee joint has been opened to show the heavy deposition of urate crystals in the articular cartilage.

Fig. 10.31 Knee joints in rheumatoid arthritis. F/63. The joints have been opened to show the gross destruction of the articular cartilages by the overgrowth of pannus. A fibrous ankylosis had occurred and the ragged appearance of the articular surfaces is partly due to the tearing of this during the opening of the joints.

Fig. 10.32 Chronic arthritis resulting from multiple haemarthroses. M/50 with haemophilia. The articular surfaces of the knee joint are markedly pitted and destroyed. The yellow pigmentation is due to the deposition of iron.

Fig. 10.32

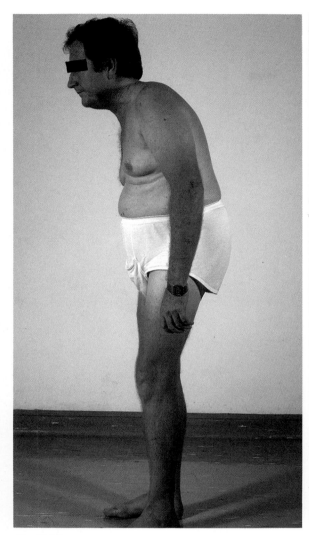

Fig. 10.33

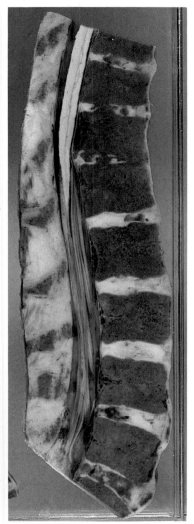

Fig. 10.34

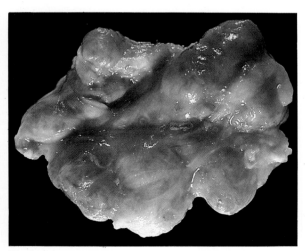

Fig. 10.35

Fig. 10.33 Ankylosing spondylitis. M/46. This man demonstrates the posture adopted to compensate for the fact that his spinal column is rigid.

Fig. 10.34 Spinal column of ankylosing spondylitis. M/50. The calcification of the interspinous ligaments is demonstrated.

Fig. 10.35 Giant cell tumour of tendon sheath (benign synovioma) excised from the finger. F/58. The tumour is lobulated and the brown colour is due to the deposition of iron. When a similar lesion occurs in the synovial membrane within a joint it is called pigmented villo-nodular synovitis.

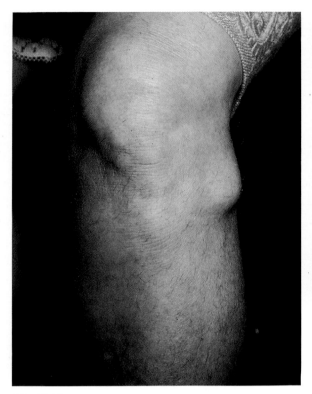

Fig. 10.37

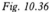

Fig. 10.36

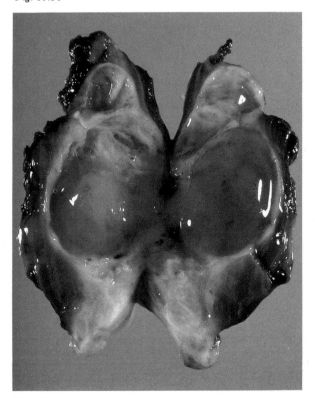

Fig. 10.38

Fig. 10.36 Cyst of the lateral meniscus of the knee. F/50.

Fig. 10.37 The lateral meniscus has been removed and the cut surface shows a multiloculated cyst containing sticky synovial fluid.

Fig. 10.38 Synovial cyst or ganglion removed from near a joint. F/52. The thin walled multiloculated cyst has been cut open. Some of the synovial fluid which it contained is still present.

Fig. 10.39 Benign subcutaneous lipoma. F/27. The cut surface shows a lobulated appearance which is accentuated by thin bands of fibrous tissue.

Fig. 10.40 Intra muscular myxoma. F/79. This tumour was removed from the right buttock. It is well circumscribed within the muscle and its cut surface shows a glistening appearance.

Fig. 10.41 Liposarcoma. M/34. The cut surface is multilobulated and contains some solid areas and some areas of haemorrhage. All malignant soft tissue tumours appear macroscopically to be well encapsulated. This leads surgeons to 'shell them out' as one would remove a pea from a pod. This invariably leaves residual tumour which will regrow if further resection is not performed.

Fig. 10.42 Rhabdomyosarcoma. F/44. This tumour was removed from the forearm with a good margin of muscle around it. The tumour has a brown colour with a central area of haemorrhage. Wide local resection wherever possible, is currently accepted as the treatment of choice for malignant soft tissue tumours.

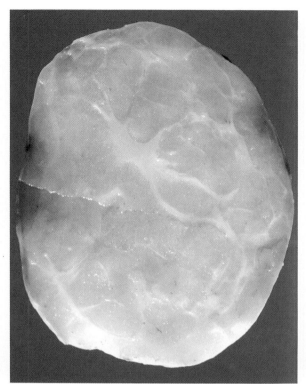

Fig. 10.39

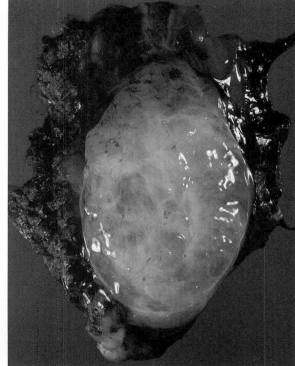

Fig. 10.40

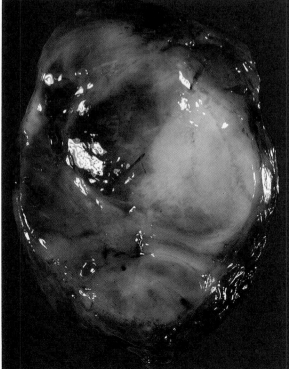

Fig. 10.41

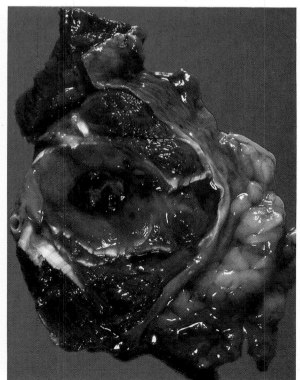

Fig. 10.42

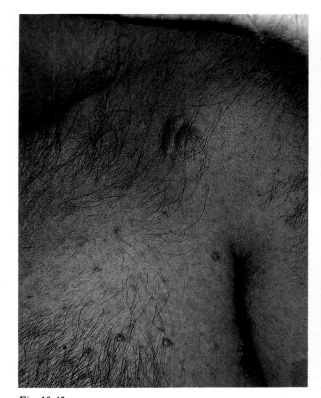

Fig. 10.43

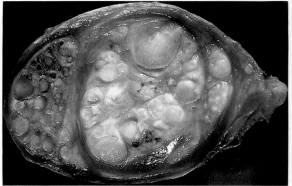

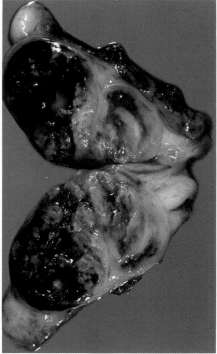

Fig. 10.46

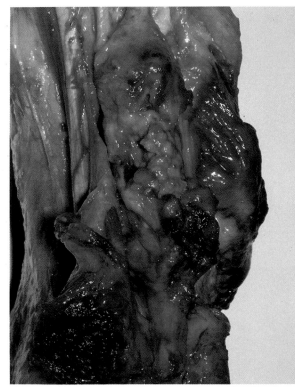

Fig. 10.45

Fig. 10.43 Neurofibromatosis. M/20. The multiple brown subcutaneous neuromata are readily visible. There is a cafe au lait spot on the inner aspect of his left arm.

Fig. 10.44 Transverse section of a plexiform neurofibroma of the sciatic nerve. M/34. This benign proliferation of nerve is often associated with this condition.

Fig. 10.45 Neurofibrosarcoma of the sciatic nerve. M/8. A large, irregular, partly necrotic tumour has developed on the sciatic nerve. Treatment was amputation of the leg. This patient had neurofibromatosis.

Fig. 10.46 Benign neurilemmoma. F/41. These tumours are usually single and their cut surface has a variegated appearance, as this one has. It is usually not associated with neurofibromatosis.

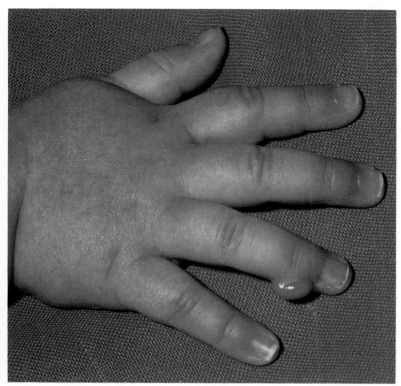

Fig. 10.47

Fig. 10.47 Digital fibroma on the third finger. F/6 months.

Fig. 10.48 Keloid scar on the shoulder. F/31.

Fig. 10.49 Keloid scar. Ear piercing is popular in many parts of the world. This is a potent cause of keloid scars.

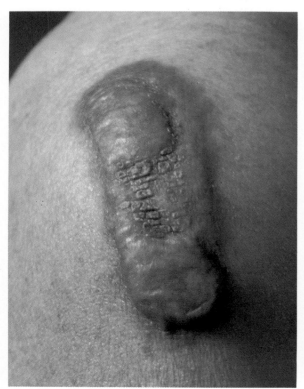

Fig. 10.48

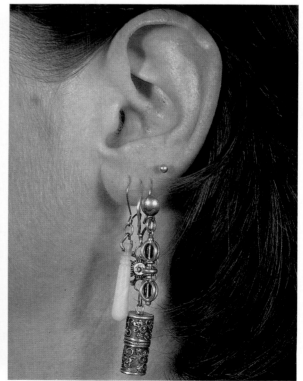

Fig. 10.49

Fig. 10.50 Plantar fibromatosis. M/12. This mass of fibrous tissue was excised from the sole of the foot. Some plantar muscle is visible in the lower portion of the specimen. This tumour is locally aggressive, and will recur if it is not completely excised.

Fig. 10.51 Dupuytren's contracture of the hand. M/50. A hard lump develops in the palm and, as it contracts, the finger is flexed towards it. The fibrous tissue in this abnormality is exactly the same as that seen in plantar fibromatosis.

Fig. 10.52 Desmoid tumour removed from the abdominal wall. M/18. The fleshy, fibrous nature of the tumour can be seen in this cross section. This is another example of a locally aggressive fibromatosis.

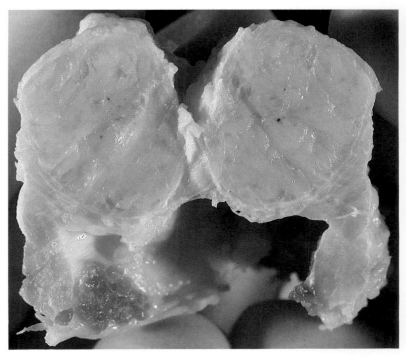

Fig. 10.50

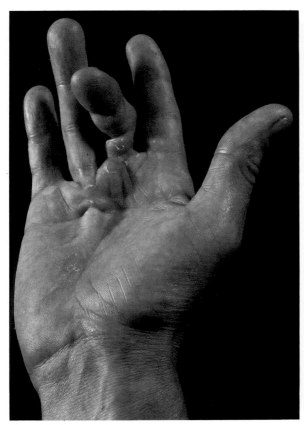

Fig. 10.51

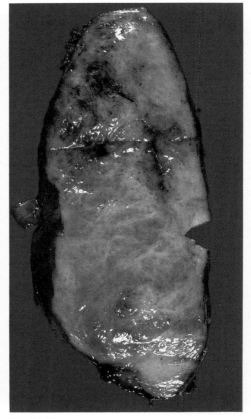

Fig. 10.52

11

Nervous system

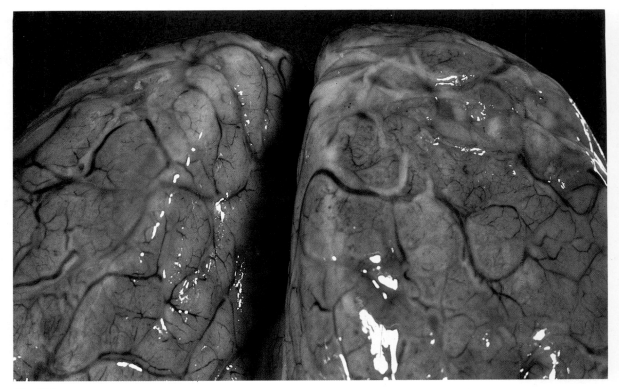

Fig. 11.1

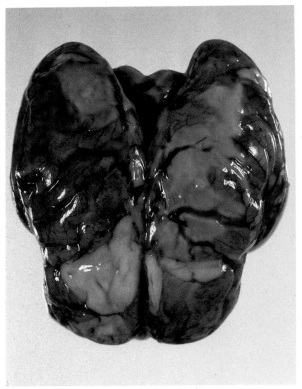

Fig. 11.2

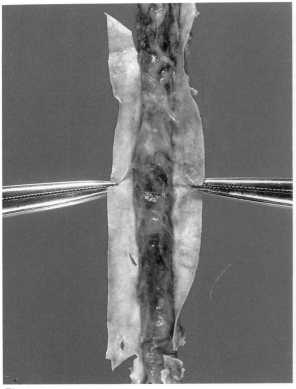

Fig. 11.3

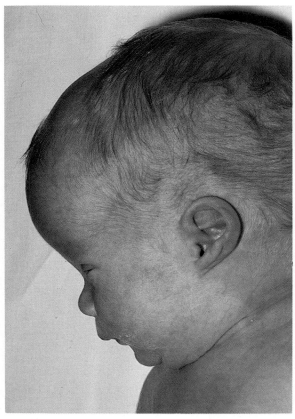

Fig. 11.4

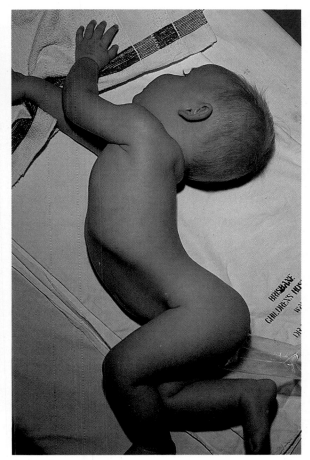

Fig. 11.5

Fig. 11.1 Acute meningitis. M/1. There are focal collections of pus in the subarachnoid space. This is the usual post mortem appearance of meningitis. Haemophilus influenzae was cultured from the CSF before death.

Fig. 11.2 Neonatal meningitis. M/4 days. The meninges are reddened from vascular congestion. Thick, greenish pus fills the subarachnoid space. Most cases of neonatal meningitis are due to coliform organisms as this one was. The leptomeninges over the frontal lobes have been torn and the surface of the brain is visible.

Fig. 11.3 Meningitis involving the spinal cord. M/3 months. The dura has been reflected and pus can be seen in the subarachnoid space. It is from this space that CSF is aspirated during lumbar puncture.

Fig. 11.4 Meningitis: bulging of the anterior fontanelle in a two month old male infant. Meningitis causes raised intracranial pressure, and this can be easily seen in a baby because of tenseness or bulging of the fontanelle.

Fig. 11.5 Meningitis causing opisthotonos. M/1. Pus in the subarachnoid space causes spasm of neck muscles giving the clinical sign of neck stiffness. In severe cases there is spasm of all the back muscles—opisthotonos.

Fig. 11.6 Meningitis: cerebro-spinal fluid obtained at lumbar puncture. From left to right: (1) xanthochromic fluid, indicating the previous presence of blood; (2) clear CSF; and (3) cloudy CSF. Cloudy CSF is presumptive evidence of meningitis.

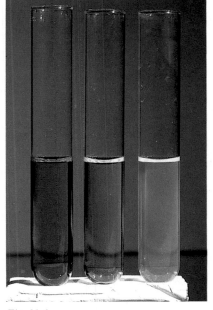

Fig. 11.6

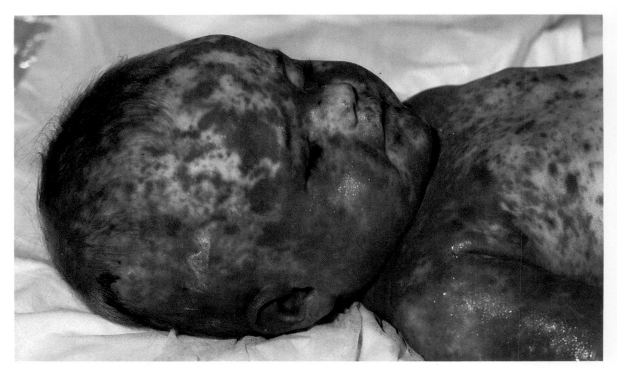

Fig. 11.7

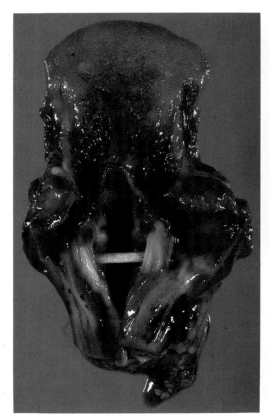

Fig. 11.8

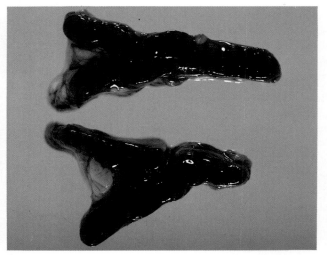

Fig. 11.9

Fig. 11.7 Waterhouse Fridericksen Syndrome. F/6 months. This child was well in the morning, became febrile and sick at mid-day, developed this red, haemorrhagic rash soon afterwards, and died in the late afternoon.

Figs. 11.8 & 11.9 Post mortem examination performed on the baby in Fig. 11.7 revealed redness of the epiglottis (Fig. 11.8) and bilateral adrenal haemorrhage (Fig. 11.9). No other abnormality was found. These are the classical features of the Waterhouse Fridericksen Syndrome which is caused most frequently by Neisseria meningitidis, but other organisms that cause meningitis may also produce the syndrome.

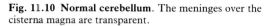

Fig. 11.10 Normal cerebellum. The meninges over the cisterna magna are transparent.

Fig. 11.11 Meningitis cerebellum. F/3 months. The meninges over the cisterna magna are opaque due to the presence of pus in the subarachnoid space. This has occluded the CSF outlets of the fourth ventricle resulting in hydrocephalus—one of the complications of meningitis.

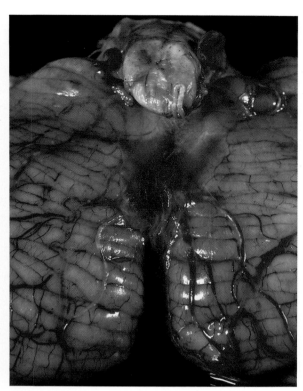

Fig. 11.10

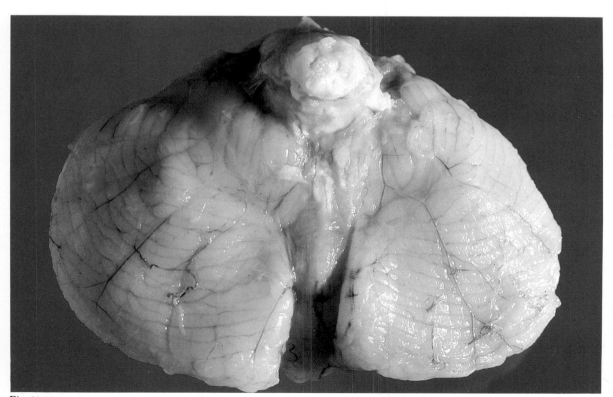

Fig. 11.11

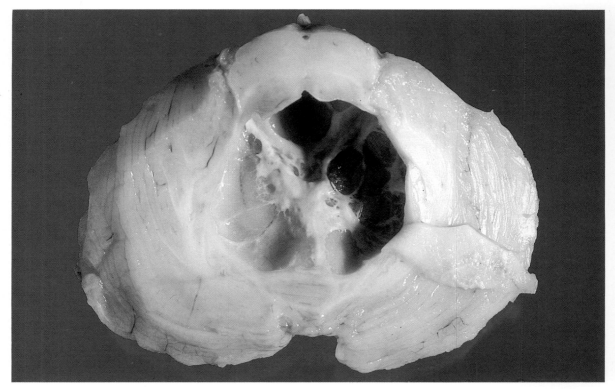

Fig. 11.12

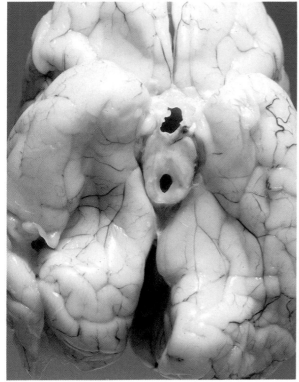

Fig. 11.13

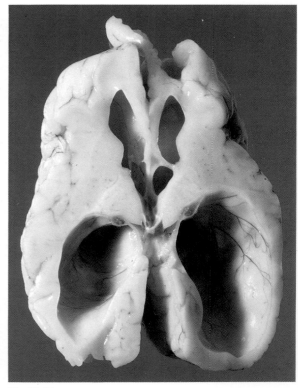

Fig. 11.14

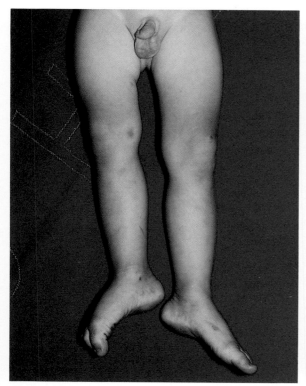

Fig. 11.15

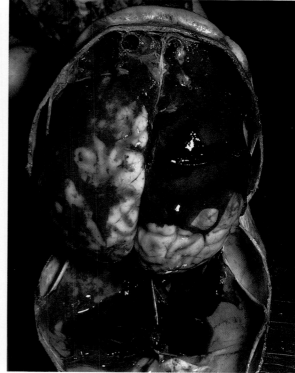

Fig. 11.16

Fig. 11.12 Meningitis hydrocephalus.
Cross-section of the cerebellum shown
in Fig. 11.11 illustrating dilatation of
the fourth ventricle with purulent
exudate attached to its lining.

Fig. 11.13 Same case showing dilatation
of the cerebral aqueduct.

Fig. 11.14 Same case showing dilatation
of the third and both lateral ventricles.

**Fig. 11.15 Meningitis complicated by
osteomyelitis.** M/2½. Shortening of the
right leg resulting from osteomyelitis of
the head of the femur following
meningitis.

Fig. 11.16 Meningitis: subdural
collection of serosanguinous fluid. F/2.
A common complication of meningitis.

Fig. 11.17 Meningitis complicated by a
cortical infarct. Neonate. Note that
neonatal brains do not have well defined
grey and white matter.

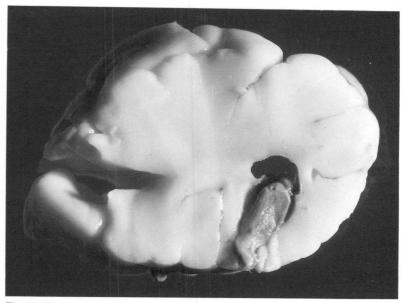

Fig. 11.17

Fig. 11.18 Tuberculous meningitis. M/39. Note the opacity of the leptomeninges covering the interpeduncular cistern. The pus tends to accumulate along the base of the brain in TB meningitis.

Fig. 11.19 Tuberculoma. M/25. There is a well circumscribed mass in the right frontal lobe. Space occupying lesions such as this are sometimes seen in patients with TB meningitis and they may present with clinical features that mimic a neoplasm.

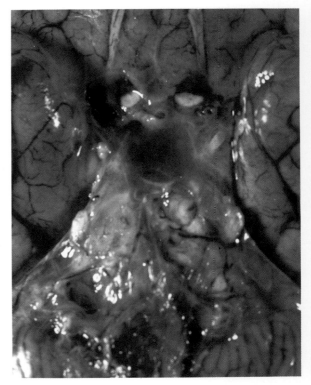

Fig. 11.18

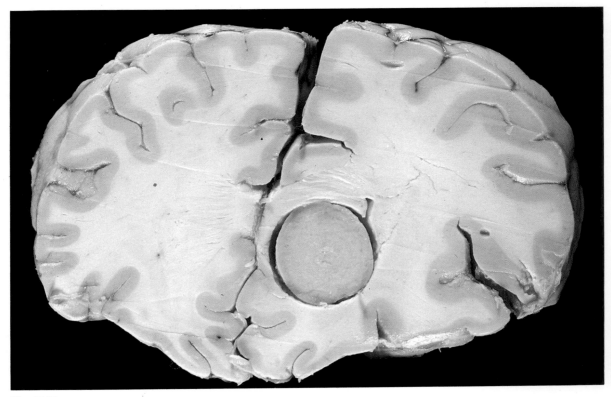

Fig. 11.19

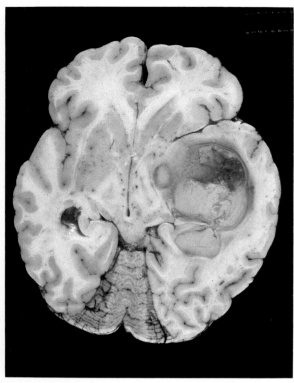

Fig. 11.20

Fig. 11.20 Cerebral abscess in the right hemisphere. M/9. The abscess has been present for some time as indicated by the presence of a partial capsule. Recent extension has occurred in two places through this capsule.

Fig. 11.21 Toruloma in the left hemisphere. M/50. Note the multiloculated and mucoid appearance of the cut surface which is fairly characteristic of this infection. Toruloma is a complication of Cryptococcal meningitis.

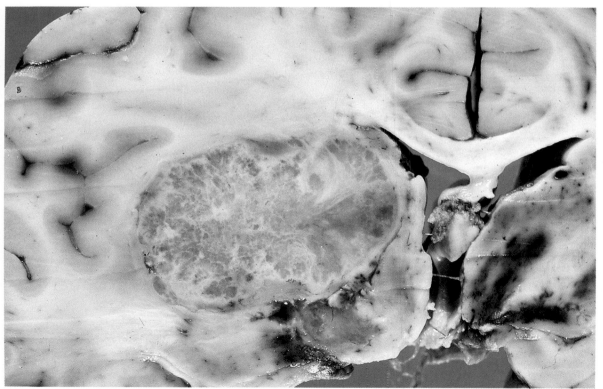

Fig. 11.21

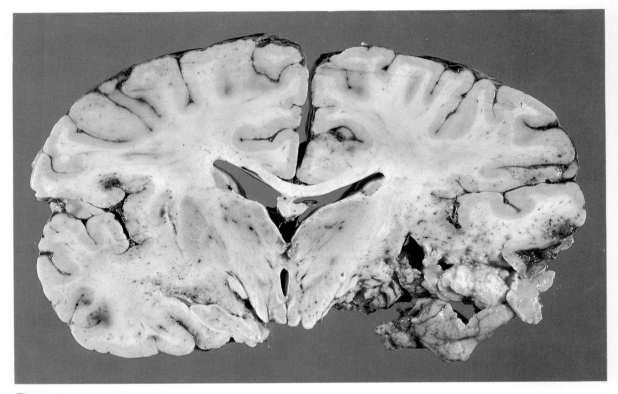

Fig. 11.22

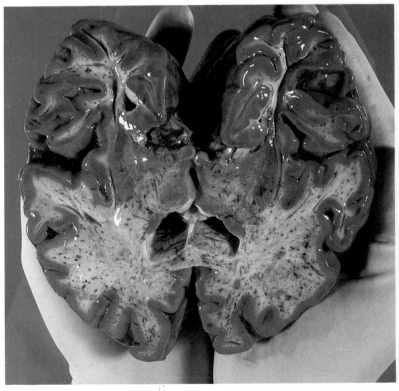

Fig. 11.22 Herpes encephalitis. M/44.
There is marked necrosis of the right
temporal lobe and petechial haemorrhages
and early necrosis in the left temporal
lobe. This distribution is characteristic of
Herpes simplex encephalitis.

Fig. 11.23 Cerebral malaria. M/67. The
patient recently returned to Australia
from Papua New Guinea, became febrile
and died before the correct diagnosis was
made. Note the multiple petechial
haemorrhages throughout the white
matter of the brain. This is the
characteristic macroscopic appearance of
this condition, but it is not present in all
cases.

Fig. 11.23

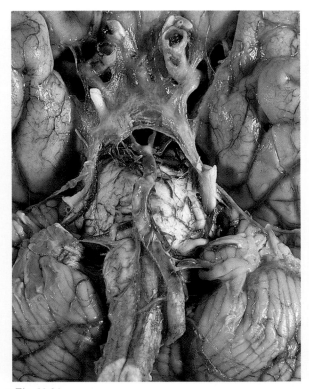

Fig. 11.24

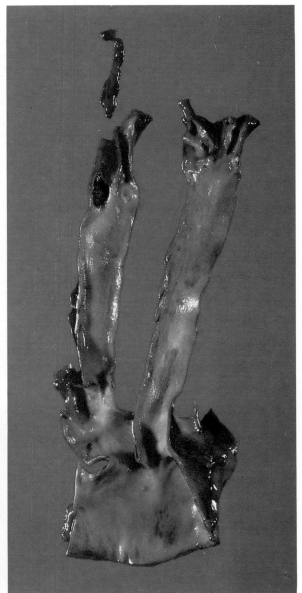

Fig. 11.25

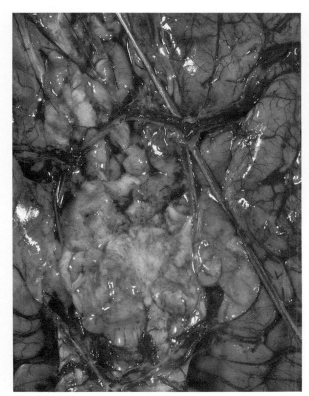

Fig. 11.26

Fig. 11.24 Cerebral infarction. Thrombosis of the left internal carotid artery. In passing, note the congenital absence of the right vertebral artery.

Fig. 11.25 Recent thrombosis of the right internal carotid artery at its origin in the neck. F/30.

Fig. 11.26 Recent thrombosis of the left middle cerebral artery. F/82.

Fig. 11.27 Cerebral infarction. M/60. Recent infarction in the distribution of the right middle cerebral artery which could have been caused by thrombosis at any of the sites illustrated in Figs. 11.24–11.26. There is haemorrhage into the anterior portion of the infarct and the temporal lobe is soft and swollen.

Fig. 11.28 Coronal section of brain showing haemorrhagic infarction in the distribution of the right middle cerebral artery. M/48.

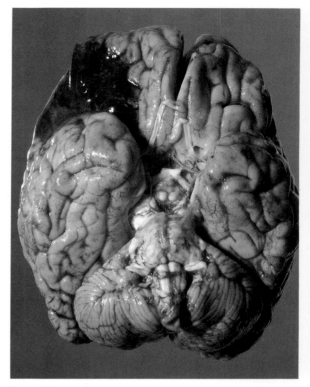

Fig. 11.27

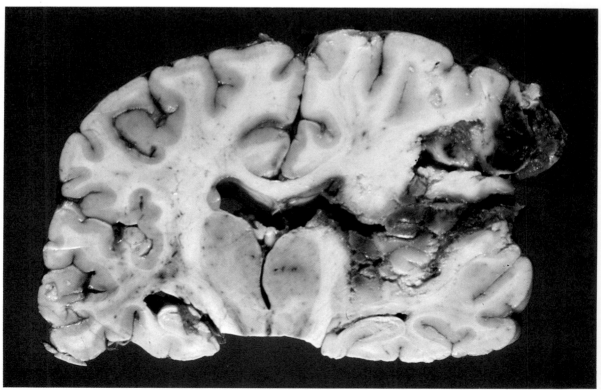

Fig. 11.28

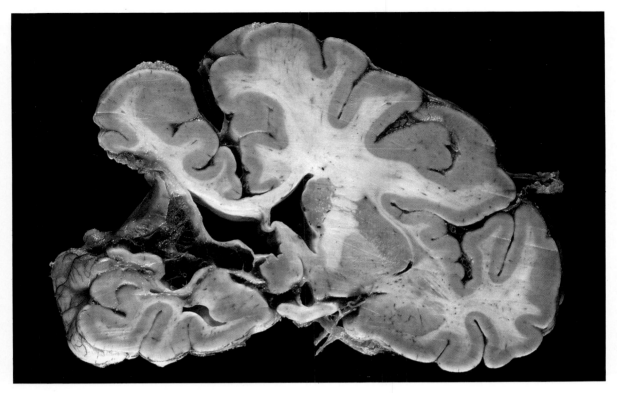

Fig. 11.29

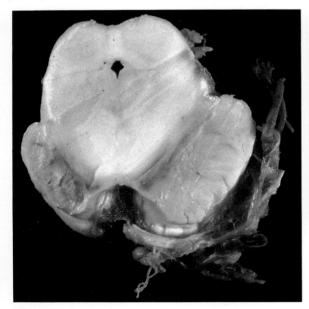

Fig. 11.30

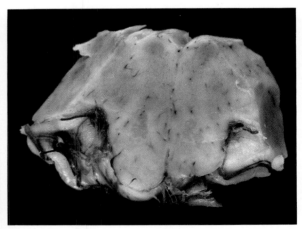

Fig. 11.31

Fig. 11.29 Cerebral infarction. Old infarction in the distribution of the left middle cerebral artery. F/59. The necrotic brain substance has liquefied leaving a cyst.

Fig. 11.30 Atrophy of the left cerebral peduncle from the brain in Fig. 11.29.

Fig. 11.31 Atrophy of the right pyramidal tract from the brain in Fig. 11.29.

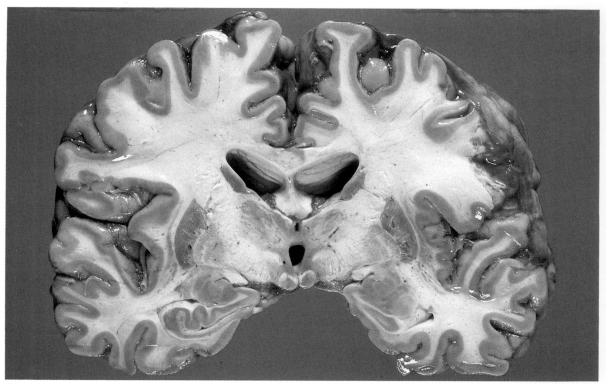

Fig. 11.32

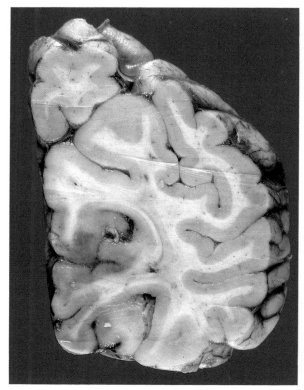

Fig. 11.33

Fig. 11.34

Fig. 11.32 Infarction of specific areas of the brain. Infarction of a localised area of cortex and underlying white matter at the postero-inferior end of the left frontal lobe—the motor speech area. F/78.

Fig. 11.33 Recent infarction of the medial aspect of the right occipital lobe due to occlusion of the right posterior cerebral artery. F/69. This caused blurring of her vision.

Fig. 11.34 Cystic area in the distribution of the left posterior cerebral artery. M/77. The result of an old infarct.

Fig. 11.35 Vertebro-basilar insufficiency. Recent thrombosis of the basilar artery. M/55. Note the infarction in the pons.

Fig. 11.36 Recent infarction in the distribution of the right posterior inferior cerebellar artery. M/53. This artery arises from the basilar, and thrombosis of the basilar results in infarction of the brain stem and frequently the inferior surface of the cerebellum as well.

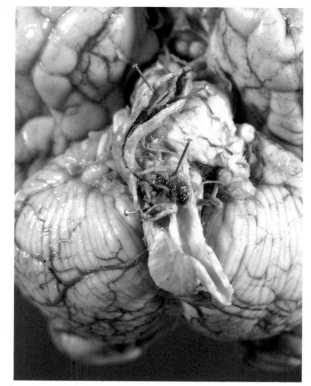

Fig. 11.35

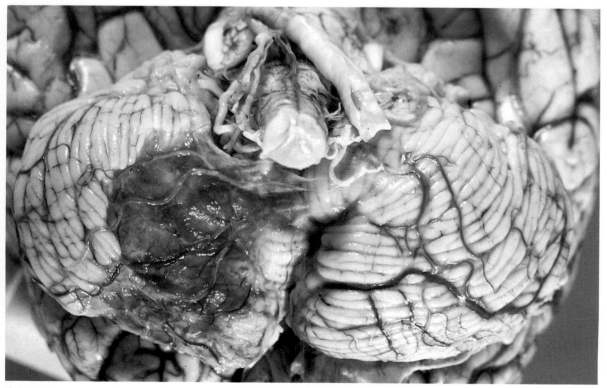

Fig. 11.36

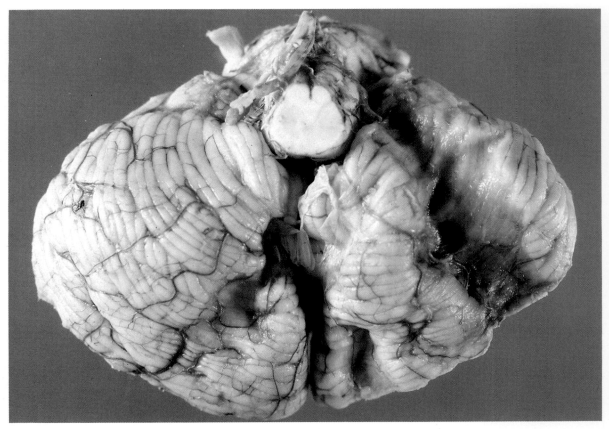

Fig. 11.37

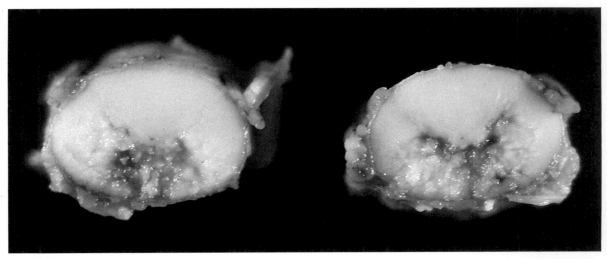

Fig. 11.38

Fig. 11.37 Vertebro-basilar insufficiency. Old infarction in the distribution of both posterior inferior cerebellar arteries. F/54.

Fig. 11.38 Recent infarction of the anterior portion of the spinal cord. M/83. This occurred as a result of thrombosis of the anterior spinal artery.

Fig. 11.39 Neonatal intracranial haemorrhage.
Intraventricular haemorrhage resulting from hypoxia. M/3
weeks. The brain shows almost complete absence of
development of gyri, indicating marked prematurity.

Fig. 11.40 Tear in the tentorium cerebelli which resulted from
traumatic delivery and caused death from haemorrhage.

Fig. 11.41 Fat embolus. F/25. The patient was in a
motorcycle accident and sustained multiple fractures of both
legs. The fat emboli caused petechial haemorrhages in the
white matter throughout the brain resulting in coma and death.

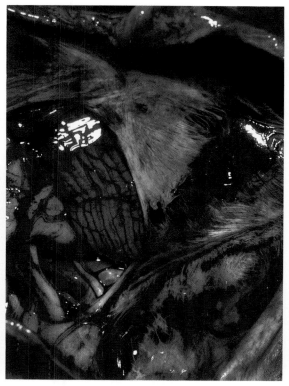

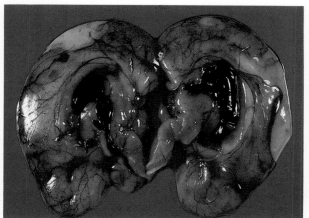

Fig. 11.39

Fig. 11.40

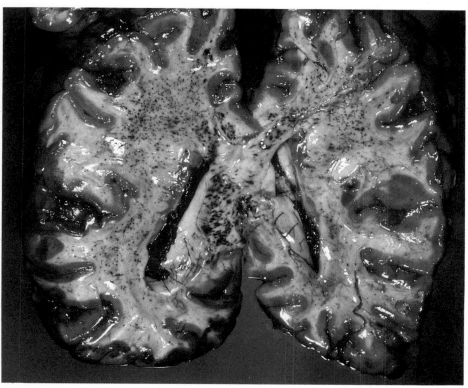

Fig. 11.41

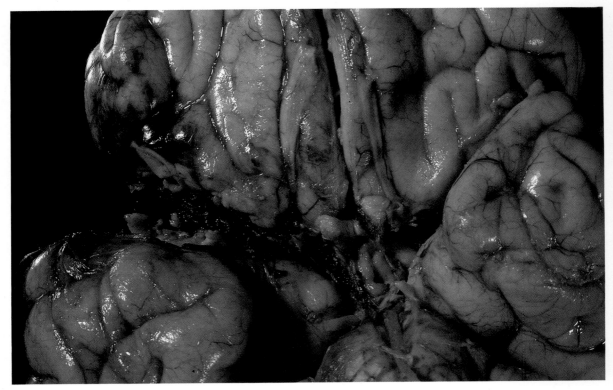

Fig. 11.42

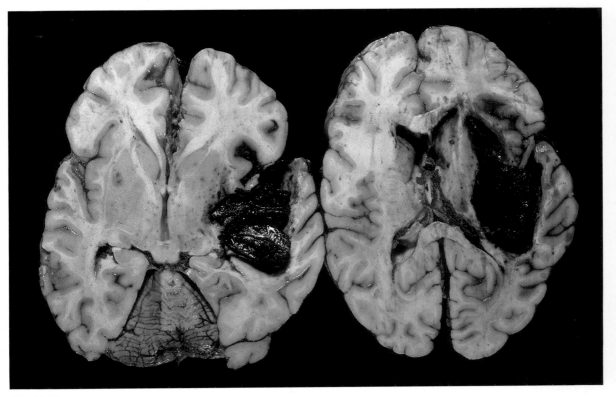

Fig. 11.43

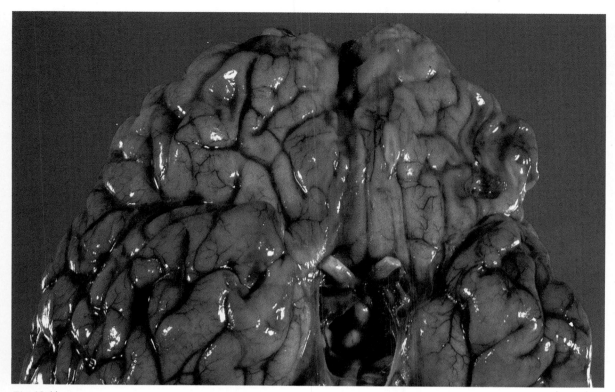

Fig. 11.44

Fig. 11.42 Mycotic embolus occluding the right middle
cerebral artery. M/13 with bacterial endocarditis.

Fig. 11.43 Cut slices of the brain in Fig. 11.42 showing
intracerebral haemorrhage resulting from rupture of the
mycotic aneurysm which developed in the middle cerebral
artery.

Fig. 11.44 Traumatic brain damage. Undersurface of the
brain showing areas of old necrosis and haemorrhage as shown
by the brown staining of the meninges covering the anterior
surfaces of frontal and temporal lobes and the inferior surfaces
of the frontal lobes. M/60. These represent areas of damage
caused by acceleration/deceleration injury to the brain.

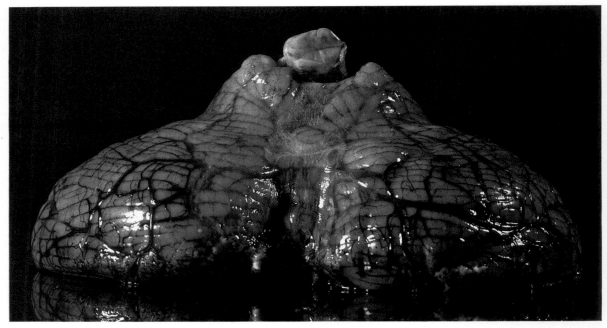

Fig. 11.45

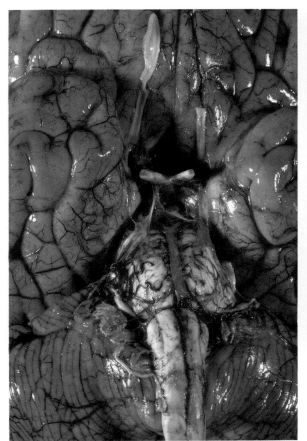

Fig. 11.46

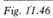
Fig. 11.47

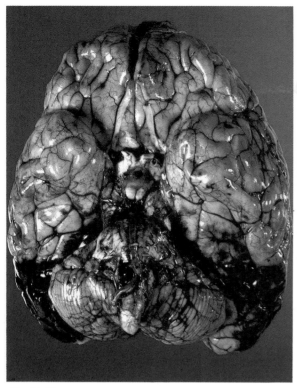

Fig. 11.48

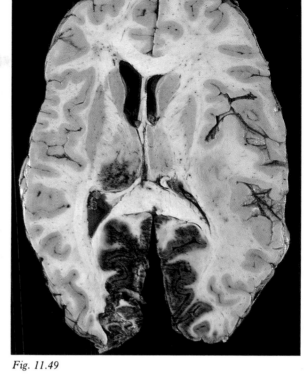

Fig. 11.49

Fig. 11.45 Effects of raised intracranial pressure. Tonsillar herniation of the cerebellum. The groove made by the foramen magnum can be seen. There had been increased intracranial pressure and this forced the cerebellar tonsils through the foramen magnum causing pressure on the brain stem—'coning'.

Fig. 11.46 Uncal herniation. The same brain as in Fig. 11.45. The brain is viewed on its under surface and the left uncus is more prominent than the right. It has herniated medially, causing stretching of the posterior communicating artery, and would have caused stretching of the sixth nerve as well.

Fig. 11.47 Multiple brain stem haemorrhages. Another complication of raised intracranial pressure and frequently the final cause of death.

Fig. 11.48 Recent infarction of both occipital lobes due to occlusion of both posterior cerebral arteries caused by compression of the arteries against the free border of the tentorium cerebelli by raised intracranial pressure.

Fig. 11.49 Coronal section of the brain showing the distribution of this infarction.

Fig. 11.50 Infarction of the cerebral peduncles which are also supplied by small branches of the posterior cerebral arteries.

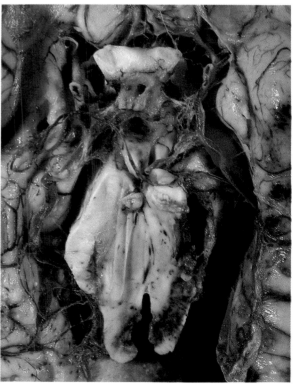

Fig. 11.50

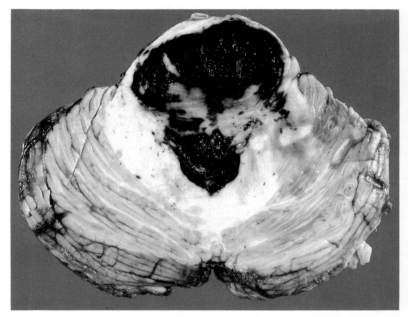

Fig. 11.61

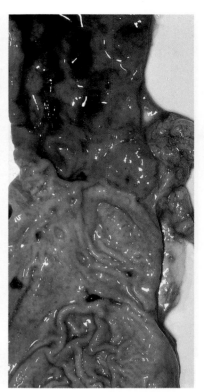

Fig. 11.63

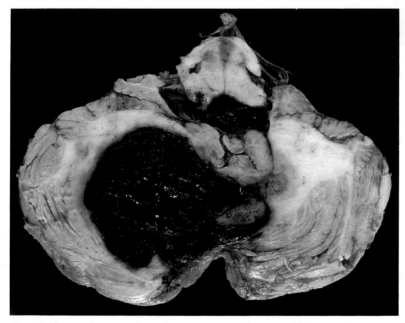

Fig. 11.62

Fig. 11.61 Haemorrhage: pontine. F/42. Hypertension.

Fig. 11.62 Intracerebellar haemorrhage. M/50. Hypertension.
This is the least common type of hypertensive haemorrhage.

Fig. 11.63 Acute gastric erosions, a well recognised
complication of intracerebral haemorrhage. M/57.

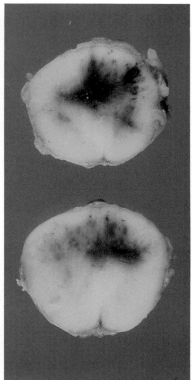

Fig. 11.65

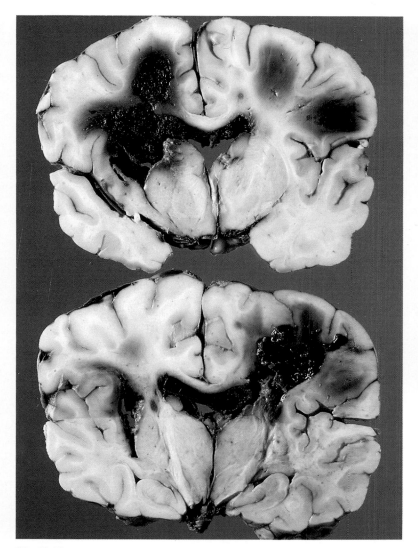

Fig. 11.64

Fig. 11.64 Multiple haemorrhages throughout both hemispheres. F/16. The patient had acute myeloblastic leukemia and died as a result of bleeding diathesis. The fact that the haemorrhages are multiple indicates a bleeding disorder rather than rupture of a major vessel.

Fig. 11.65 Haemorrhage into the spinal cord resulting from a road traffic accident. M/61.

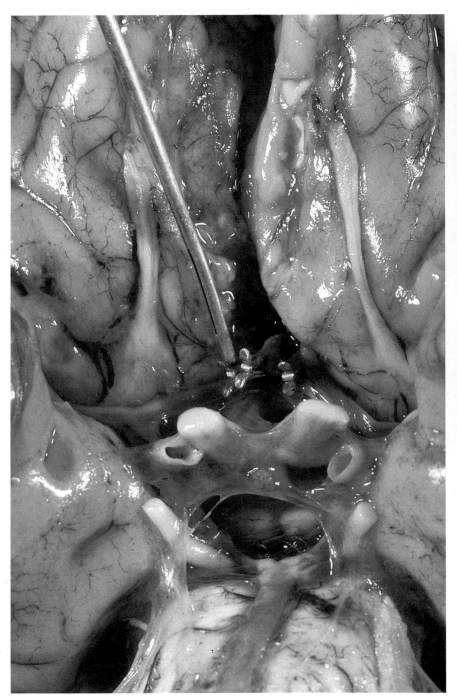

Fig. 11.66

Fig. 11.67

Fig. 11.66 Berry aneurysm on the anterior communicating artery. M/48. The aneurysm bled, causing **subarachnoid haemorrhage**. Surgical clips were applied to the base of the aneurysm to control the bleeding.

Fig. 11.67 Subarachnoid haemorrhage in the spinal cord following rupture of a berry aneurysm. F/35.

Fig. 11.68 Ruptured aneurysm on the right internal carotid artery at the point where it becomes the middle cerebral artery. It had caused subarachnoid haemorrhage and had extended into the optic nerve. F/57.

Fig. 11.69 Large unruptured aneurysm of the basilar artery, an incidental finding. F/61.

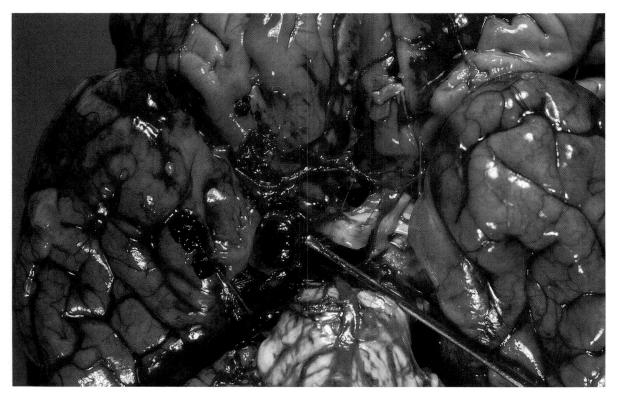

Fig. 11.68

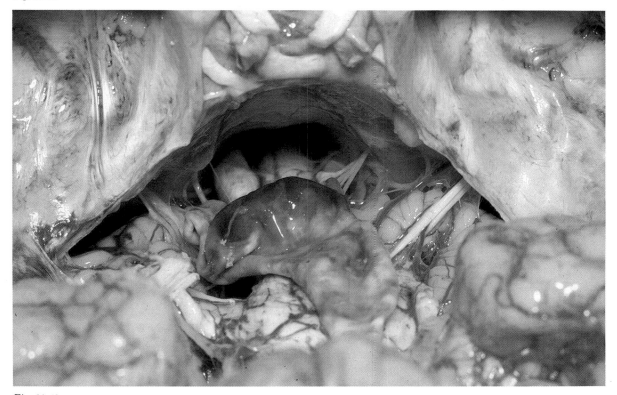

Fig. 11.69

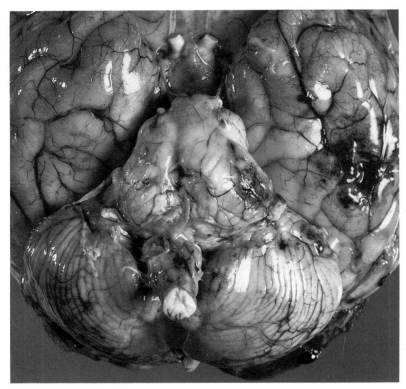

Fig. 11.74 Astrocytoma in the brain stem. F/8. Note the grossly enlarged pons. These tumours occur particularly in children and are relatively slowly growing.

Fig. 11.75 Transverse section of pons and cerebellum showing haemorrhage into a pontine astrocytoma. M/15.

Fig. 11.76 Astrocytoma. Skull irregularly thinned by raised intracranial pressure caused by the presence of the tumour. F/3. This appearance is sometimes called the 'beaten copper' skull.

Fig. 11.77 Cerebellum containing a large astrocytoma. F/6. The majority of brain tumours in children occur below the tentorium cerebelli.

Fig. 11.74

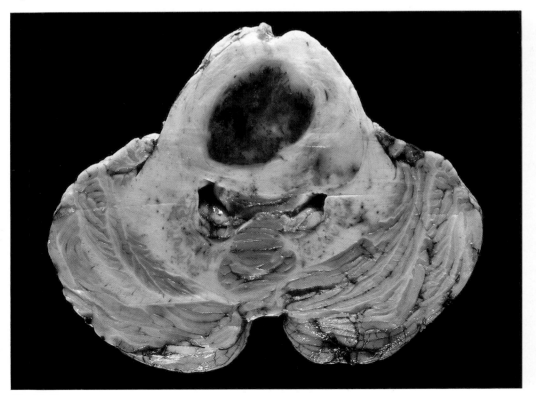

Fig. 11.75

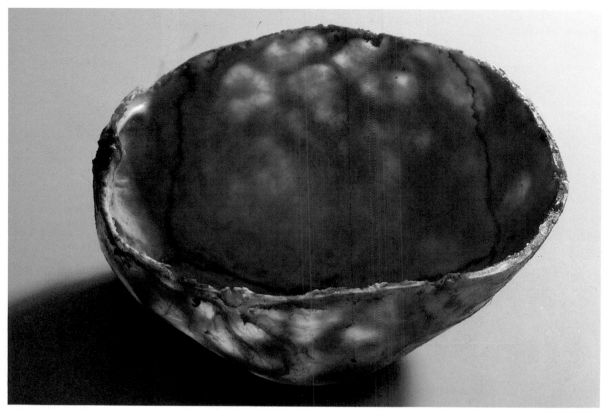

Fig. 11.76

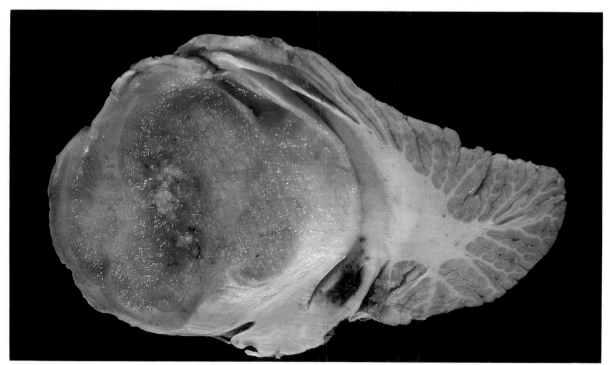

Fig. 11.77

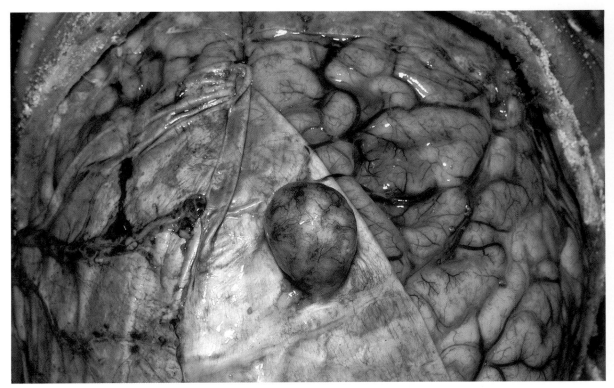

Fig. 11.82

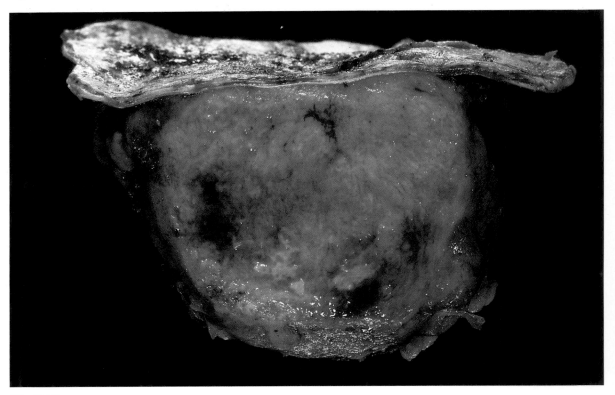

Fig. 11.83

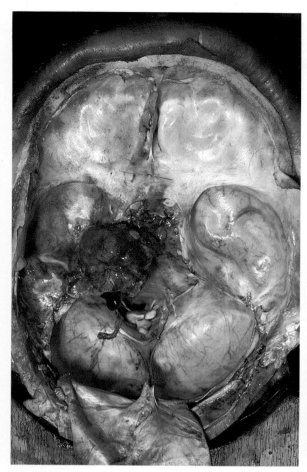

Fig. 11.84

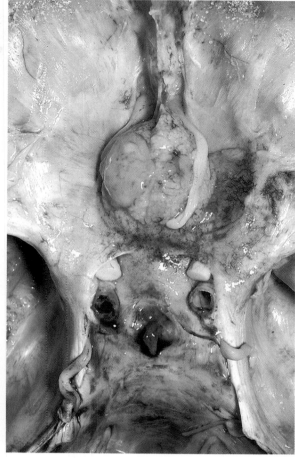

Fig. 11.85

Fig. 11.82 Meningioma. Small, asymptomatic tumour attached to the dura. F/46.

Fig. 11.83 Transverse section of a meningioma removed surgically together with the attached dura. M/78.

Fig. 11.84 The brain has been removed to demonstrate the presence of a meningioma attached to the left petrous temporal bone and impinging on the pitúitary fossa. M/70.

Fig. 11.85 Meningioma arising from the olfactory groove. Incidental post mortem finding. M/89.

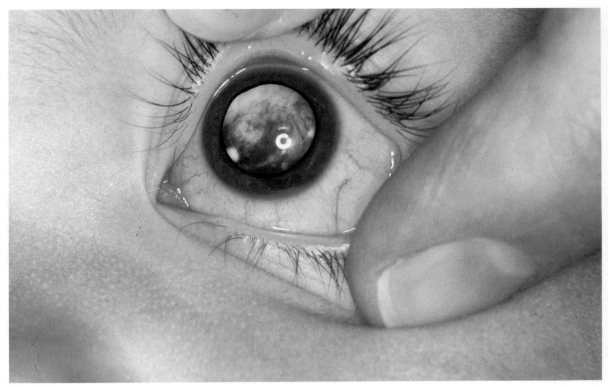

Fig. 11.86

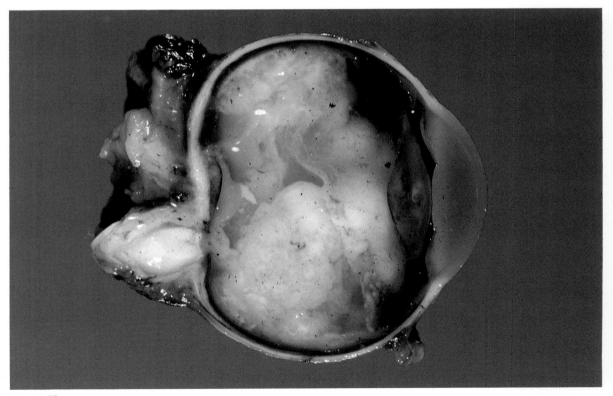

Fig. 11.87

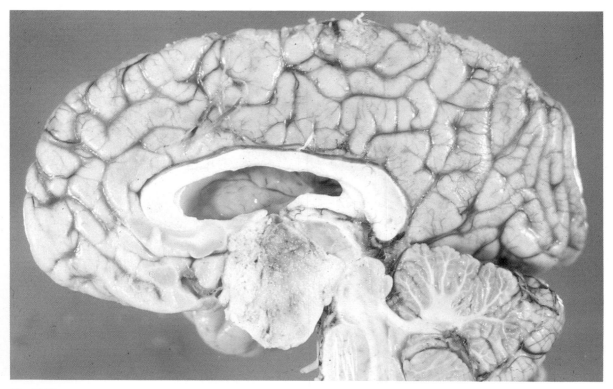

Fig. 11.88

Fig. 11.86 Retinoblastoma. F/2. The mother was alerted to the condition by the white colour of the pupil. There was also some loss of vision.

Fig. 11.87 Retinoblastoma filling the posterior chamber of the eye removed surgically. There was no spread along the subdural space around the optic nerve, no tumour in the other eye, and no family history—features that are often present.

Fig. 11.88 Large pituitary adenoma. F/12. Microscopically this was a chromophobe adenoma and clinically it was causing local pressure effects.

Fig. 11.89 Craniopharyngioma in the pituitary fossa. F/52. The main bulk of the tumour was situated above the sella.

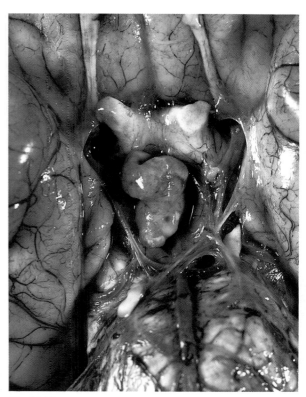

Fig. 11.89

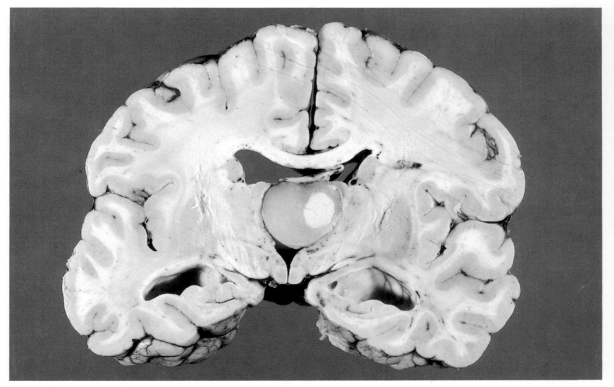

Fig. 11.90

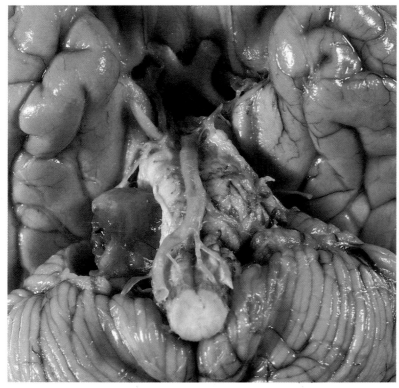

Fig. 11.91

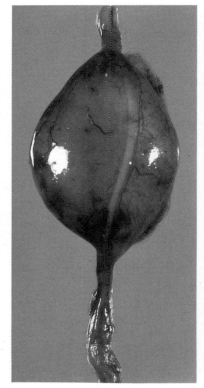

Fig. 11.92

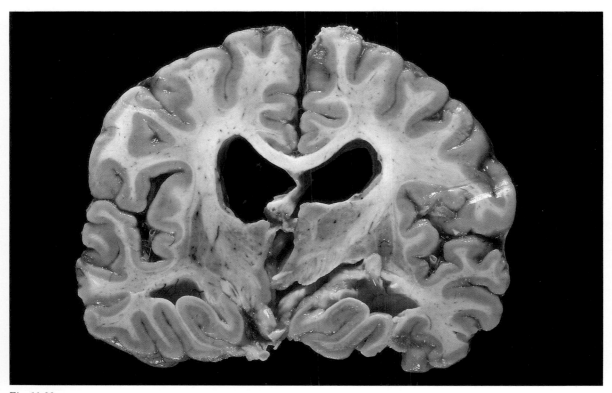

Fig. 11.93

Fig. 11.90 Colloid cyst of the third ventricle. M/16. The patient presented with intermittent headaches particularly in the head down position. Lumbar puncture was performed in a country hospital and the pressure shift resulted in herniation of the cerebellar tonsils (coning) and death.

Fig. 11.91 Neurilemmoma (acoustic neuroma) arising from the right eighth. nerve. M/50. An incidental post mortem finding. It usually presents as deafness.

Fig. 11.92 Neurilemmoma arising on a peripheral nerve. M/20. Presented as a subcutaneous tumour which was excised.

Fig. 11.93 Huntington's Chorea. F/54. Note the gross atrophy of both caudate nuclei and both basal ganglia. There is marked compensatory hydrocephalus resulting from the cortical and basal ganglia atrophy.

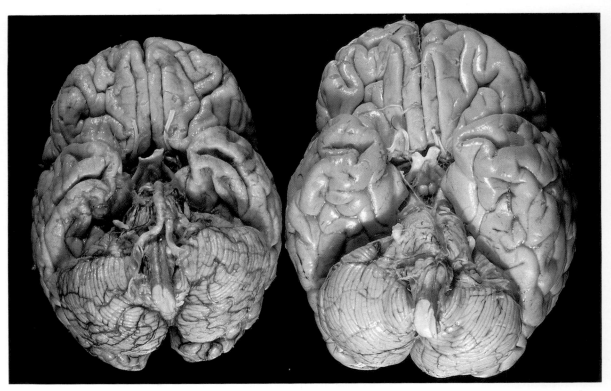

Fig. 11.94

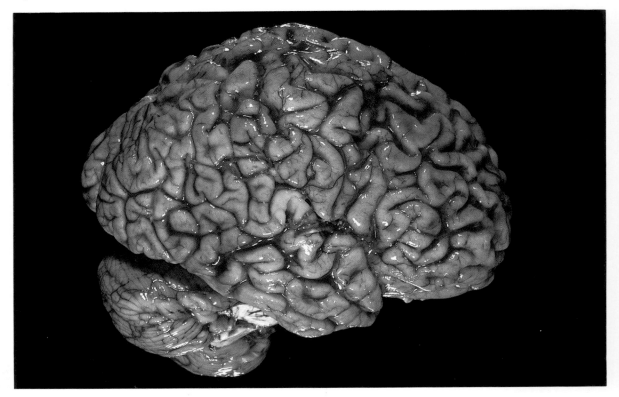

Fig. 11.95

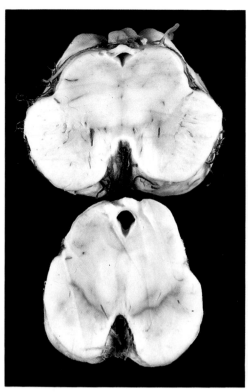

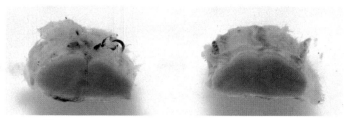

Fig. 11.97

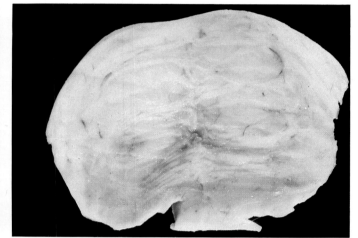

Fig. 11.96

Fig. 11.98

Fig. 11.94 Alzheimer's Disease. F/53. The atrophic brain on the left is compared with that of a normal 50 year-old on the right. Alzheimer's Disease is the commonest form of presenile dementia.

Fig. 11.95 Another case of Alzheimer's Disease. F/57. Note the gross atrophy of the cerebral gyri and widening of the sulci in all lobes but being particularly noticeable in the frontal lobe.

Fig. 11.96 Parkinson's Disease. M/65. The transverse section of the cerebral peduncles in the upper specimen shows loss of pigment in the substantia nigra. The lower specimen for comparison shows normal substantia nigra.

Fig. 11.97 Atrophy of the posterior columns of the spinal cord. Three conditions cause this appearance: Tabes dorsalis; Vitamin B12 deficiency (subacute combined degeneration); and Friedreich's ataxia.

Fig. 11.98 Central pontine myelinolysis. M/61. The area of demyelination is shown as a brownish discolouration. The patient was an alcoholic. This condition was first described in alcoholics, but it is now known to be associated with hypokalaemia, especially when this has been rapidly corrected.

Fig. 11.99 Multiple sclerosis. M/33. This diagnosis was made six years before death when the patient first complained of ataxia. The ataxia was followed by increasing weakness of legs and arms. For a few years before death from pneumonia he was confined to a wheel chair. This brain slice shows a large grey area of demyelination in the characteristic periventricular distribution. There is another large area of demyelination in the white matter of the temporal lobe.

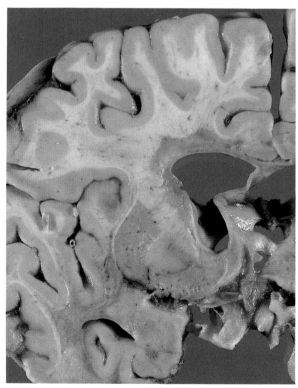

Fig. 11.99

Fig. 11.115 Poliomyelitis. Young adult male in Papua New Guinea with a withered left leg. This was a comon sight throughout the world before the introduction of the Polio vaccine.

Fig. 11.116 End stage of muscle disease. Transverse section from the atrophic muscle of a patient who had poliomyelitis as a child and died from other pathology. Note the small amount of red muscle remaining. Most of the muscle has been replaced by fat. All chronic muscle diseases progress to grossly atrophic muscle such as this. The diagnosis of primary muscle disease depends on the clinical assessment and microscopic examination of biopsies taken from muscles which are not completely atrophic.

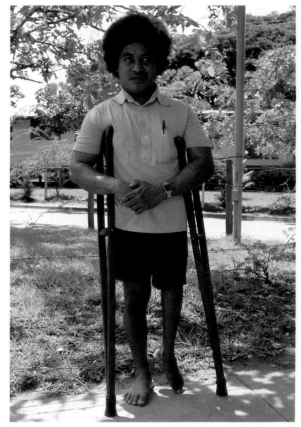

Fig. 11.115

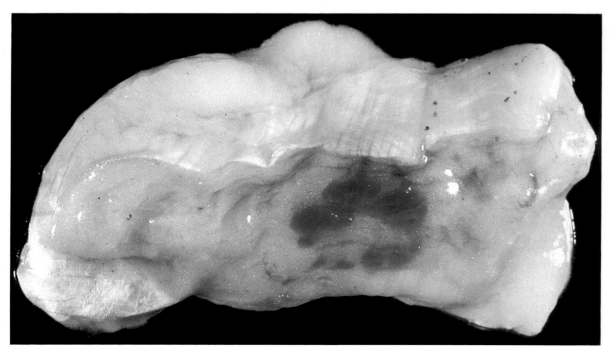

Fig. 11.116

Index